D1017038

Metamorphosis:
Transforming Your Body, Mind & Life!

Join the Wellness Revolution!

- **Use leading-edge science and modern, enlightened mentoring to help you rejuvenate your mind and sculpt your body.**
- **Stop runaway stress in its tracks and reverse its damages.**
- **Reclaim that "youth inside" for a healthier, fitter, more vibrant you!**

Charles Webb, DC, CCST

With Don Elefante, Researcher, Editor-in-Chief

Metamorphosis:
Transforming Your Body, Mind & Life!
Dr. Charles S. Webb, DC, CCST

July 2011

Revised and expanded edition of:
Reclaim 24: Quickly Reclaim Your Health, Your Youth, & Your Life

Copyright 2008–2011 by Charles S. Webb, DC

ISBN-13: 978-0-9846478-0-4

BookMasters, Inc.
30 Amberwood Parkway
Ashland, OH 44805

www.bookmasters.com

Contents

Contents (cont)

A Few Words from Those Who Know Something about Metamorphosis!

"Recently, I went to my doctor for my annual physical and she was really amazed at the lab results. The glucose, liver enzymes, the weight, all the negative indications have gone down. She was amazed – what did I do? So I told her about the Wellness coaching that I've been receiving from Dr. Webb and his doctors and she was just really happy about the results. And by my medical records I actually lost 24 pounds."

Ruffino Navalta
San Antonio, TX

"I'm a big guy, but so are the guys I'm wrestling ... and they're not so nice in the ring!

"The only way I could stay in the ring against these Giants was to keep in the best shape possible.

"Thanks to Dr. Webb and his Lifestyle program, I was not only able to stay in the ring, but ultimately won the World Champion Title."

Lance Cade
World Wrestling Champion

Acknowledgements

So many people deserve thanks for seeing me through this project, especially my wife, Mindi, who gave her trust and support from the moment of conception. I also thank my two beautiful children, Amanda and Landon, for inspiring purpose in my life. I hope this book creates wellness and longevity in theirs.

I owe much gratitude to my father for teaching me about sacrifice and for all the time he set aside to be a part of my life. Thanks to my mother for showing me the power of love and friendship. Thanks to both of you for helping to sculpt me and for teaching me to believe in myself.

On the business side, I'd like to thank my editor, patient, and friend, Don Elefante, whose depth of knowledge and passion for this project earned my deepest respect. I was blessed with not only an editor but also an advisor who painstakingly labored behind the scenes, never ceasing from start to finish. Don worked on the first edition of this book, *Reclaim 24*. Starting with my original draft, he helped to fill in the gaps and delicately unwound a multitude of complex concepts that might have otherwise confused readers. The second edition, *Metamorphosis,* is the result of an additional four years of research and clinical experience. We both recognized the importance of getting this new information into the hands of the public. I credit Don with the additional content, clarification, and reorganization that sets *Metamorphosis* apart from *Reclaim 24*. In addition, he has been a huge contributor to the expansive research that is always demanded in such undertakings.

I have many dear friends who support and show confidence in me. They know who they are. They have been wonderful sources of inspiration. My gratitude exceeds the limitations of this acknowledgements page. I must also recognize the key mentors I've had in my life. In particular, Steve Reeves for that initial glimpse into the world of sculptured physiques that inspired me to want to be my best. Thanks to every spiritual teacher and business leader who helped to mold my inner world and subsequently my outer: Wayne Dyer for first introducing me to the laws of creativity through disciplined thought; James Allen for his masterpiece, *As A Man Thinketh;* Maxwell Maltz for his systemized approach to mastering the mind; and all of the leaders introduced to me through the Nightingale-Conant corporation.

I couldn't have written this book without the dedication and health research of others who came before me and shared their discoveries. I've been honored to study with some of the best doctors in the country and continue to learn from their hard work. Because they put most of their waking hours into their passion, they have given all of us ways to find answers to reclaiming and retaining our vitality well into advanced age. In this respect I must give special thanks to researcher and personal mentor, Dr. Datis Kharrazian.

Dr. Kharrazian collaborated with me in the development and writing of Chapter 14, *The Role of Hormones in Wellness,* which is a must-read for anyone unwilling to succumb to the physical, mental, and emotional stressors that time and a fast-paced lifestyle press upon us. Few become so completely enthralled in their interests and vision that they burst forth as the best in their field, as Dr. Kharrazian has. I owe him so many thanks for stepping out of the mold and bringing receptive doctors healthy, practical and effective solutions for resolving hormonal imbalances and restoring wellness. My growing knowledge of hormonal dysfunctions, and the powerful effects that correcting them has in achieving maximum wellness, began with Dr. Kharrazian.

Above all, I consider myself a spiritual being willing and ready to make life a little bit smoother for those whose paths cross mine. I wouldn't have been able to complete this project without the divine support that comes through the inner channels of those who welcome and honor God's gifts of inspiration and insight. Indeed, I am greatly blessed.

Foreword

By the time I hadenjoyed a dozen or so visits to Dr. Webb's wellness center, we found ourselves discussing many topics of common interest. Indeed, we were compatible on many levels. That's when I learned he had written the first draft of a book describing his tried-and-true body-transformation system that he now calls Reclaim 24™. But the project languished, as book-length manuscripts often do when one is subject to the demands of research, ongoing education, family responsibilities, and a day job that often stretches into nights and weekends.

As a wellness fanatic who launched a new career in copywriting and consulting after retiring as an R&D chief information officer, I offered to help with his first book. We clicked—and here's the second edition. The evolution from the first to the second edition has been dramatic. It has captured recent and stunning scientific discoveries on diet, exercise, and the hormonal intricacies of energy metabolism and fat-burning.

Dr. Webb is a natural-born mentor who thrills at teaching people how to fend for themselves in the often mind-boggling worlds of health, fitness, and general wellness. It's so tiring to hear the same old, hackneyed advice: Eat a balanced diet from the "food pyramid," (most recently the "food plate") get regular exercise, and live a life of moderation. But look around at all the obese and sick people taking handfuls of costly lifetime drugs, giving up body parts to the surgeon's knife, and watching their vitality and quality of life go down the tubes day by day. Something is wrong! And it just keeps getting worse.

What differentiates Dr. Webb's approach from the norm is that he provides a connect-the-dots, five-pillar *system* that people can tailor to their busy lifestyles. For those willing to take charge of their own destinies, his easy-to-follow system rides on a foundation of scientific research that hasn't been mangled by lobbies, special interests, or government bureaucrats. Moreover, he's out there with myth-busting guns ablazing. I like that! Too many enlightened medical and health professionals are not saying what needs to be said for fear of censure—or worse. They wince under the menacing crush of three-letter acronyms. Who can blame them?

Embrace what's in these pages if you want to reclaim and hold onto more of the youth and wellness that have been slipping from your grasp. It's science, not hype—and it works.

–DON ELEFANTE, EDITOR-IN-CHIEF

More Words from Those Who Know …

"I was 25 to 30 lbs. over my ideal weight, I had high blood pressure, I was on hypertension medication, I had a high fasting blood glucose level that put me in a type II diabetes range, and high triglycerides and cholesterol.

"In only six weeks of following Dr. Webb's program I am now down to my ideal weight, I am now off of my high blood pressure medications (I'm now well below 120/70), my fasting blood glucose is around 85, well within range, and my triglycerides and cholesterol are also within range."

> John Gillespie
> Hydrologist, USAF
> San Antonio, TX

"When I began, with some skepticism, Dr. Webb's treatment for my serious needs, I listed five concerns. The first was pain, then difficulty walking, and extreme fatigue. The pain was constant and debilitating, causing depression and near despair. There was serious and ugly edema which my regular physician indifferently attributed to age. Last, was being overweight.

"Today, I have cancelled an epidural for back pain because I don't have any. I walk without pain and I have greater energy and am no longer depressed.

"Remarkably, in the past week the swollen foot and ankle edema is gone! My ankles are trim, feet go into my shoes, and I am rejoicing because life is so much happier and I am feeling so much healthier. Also, I have lost 15 lbs. These improvements are real and visible.

"Dr. Webb sent me for tests that have revealed problems that could have become critical had I not known of their existence. No other doctor has bothered to do so. Dr. Webb sees you as a living wellspring that can be improved, pain can be eliminated or reduced, and the entire body function can be made better. To be aware of feeling well gives hope and optimism."

> Maria Negri
> San Antonio, TX.

1: The "Conveyor Belt to a Living Hell"– Just Say No!

It's gut-wrenching for me to see a new patient walk into my wellness center who is too far gone for me to help reverse their pain and ravaged health. Sadly, they've usually allowed too much damage to take place for too long. Oh, yes, I can usually make them more comfortable without some drugstore product clouding and numbing their senses, but I just can't get used to serving these troubled ones and their faded hopes for restored health. I'm no wimp by a long shot, yet sometimes I cry at night having examined them and listened to their stories of anguish. But it's not that they didn't have plenty of forewarning about what was to come. I use a poignant metaphor to describe it.

Imagine a creeping conveyor belt as long as the eye can see, trailing off into the horizon. Riding along on this snail-paced belt are unwitting "passengers," all with something in common: each is losing his or her quality of life with each passing mile, and each has his fingers crossed. Some have been riding the belt for decades. Some will ride for decades more!

Where are these riders headed? Where does the belt end up? It ends up at the Pits of Misery—a kind of "living hell" destination. I say this because this is what it looks like for those who finally "arrive":

- Chronic disease symptoms such as obesity, diabetes, cancer, heart/circulatory disorders.
- Female problems, prostate problems, hearing problems.
- Heart bypass scars, the horrors of Alzheimer's, endless drug side effects.
- The life-altering and often life-destroying devastation of chemotherapy.
- Brittle bones, shrunken and stooped bodies, wheelchairs, canes, walkers, motorized carts, oxygen bottles, adult diapers (plus a medical specialty designed just for "old people" called geriatrics).
- Financial ravages resulting from explosive medical fees, drug costs, and "assisted" living expenses.

Of course, there's more ... but you get the idea. Just look around you. Once these "living hell" residents are well established, they usually find relief only in death. Yet, some will linger in the pits for many years, languishing in their states of misery. Is that any way to live?

So, what can we learn from that picture? I'll tell you. The vast majority of those riding the Conveyor Belt to a Living Hell have made many, many poor health choices over a long period. The saddest thing is that most of the riders didn't even know they were making poor choices. They listened to trusted voices, but those voices were not coming from those versed in the practice of wellness. Rather, the voices were coming from those versed in sickness care and symptom-masking through drugs. Although both sickness care and drugs are necessary under certain conditions, *they are not the tools of wellness and prevention.* Shouldn't you know the difference? Shouldn't you know what approaches are best for the changing situations you will encounter over your lifetime?

> *"Where doctors before have told me there's nothing else they can do to help or have prescribed yet another pill, Dr Webb's response has been 'that's unacceptable and here's OUR plan of action!' My body has been transformed inside and out! I feel like I have a new lease on life and I am forever grateful."*
>
> Michelle Garner
> Musician, Boerne, TX

Other "trusted" voices leading our country towards a rapid decline in health have been those coming from the processed and fast-food industries. They tell us in their endless advertising and world-class marketing lingo that they are bringing good things to life. But it's not *our* lives that are reaping the good things. It's *their* lives that benefit because cheap, denatured, calorie-laden, fat-dripping, trans-fat-impregnated, chemically-adulterated, and chemically addictive products are so profitable!

Everyone is destined to leave the planet. Even us "boomers." In the end, our bodies just stop working because that's part of nature's blueprint. But my fondest vision for those I care for and about, including myself, is that we will cavort through our "senior" years with pep in our step, a twinkle in our eyes, and the joy of getting out of bed each morning under our own steam while looking deliciously to the adventures of the day.

Then, one morning we just won't wake up, or maybe we'll keel over mid-afternoon and stir no more, or just spend a few days in the hospital saying our grateful goodbyes to those whom we love. Now that's a picture I can embrace, *and one that I know is well within most people's grasp.* Yes, I'd much rather just keel over following a fulfilling, vital life than take a long, desolate ride on the Conveyor Belt to a Living Hell that dumps me into the Pits of Misery where I might wait for—maybe even hope for—nature to bid my body adieu. I'm willing to do my part to change the long-term outcome for both my loved ones and myself. Are you?

If you'd also like to live a fabulous, productive, vital, and supportive life, and then just cease to run when your time has come to move on, then you need to know much more than what comes out of medicine, pharmacology, and TV drug commercials. For example, you need to know that it's not calendar years that harm us, but accumulated stress, inactivity, and uninspired thinking! Many aging myths need to be shattered. Even the old paradigm about the effect of genetics on long-term health is being turned on its head. For example, today we know that genetics only contributes to about 3–5% of our longevity. The rest comes from lifestyle and emotional choices that regulate how our genes express themselves under the conditions we hand them. The new field of study called *epigenetics* is involved here.

Hope Isn't the Answer

You also need to know that hope is unlikely to keep you from needing a walker, diapers, or worse as the years pass. Remember the passengers riding on the conveyor belt with their fingers crossed? Just look around you. There is plenty of hope going on, yes? But it sure doesn't seem to be helping much. Instead of hoping, you need to learn about the practice of wellness in its four key categories: physical, emotional, mental, and spiritual. Further, you need to learn that the practice of *maximum* wellness eventually requires about 95% self-care, *the type of care that can't be passed off to doctors!* If we want to break loose from the sickness paradigm, we must take personal control of our lives. Period. That is step one of the metamorphosis we desire.

Of course, we must slow down a bit as the years pass. Common sense tells us how. And we have to spend more time and resources on prevention and rejuvenation than we did in our 20's because stress damage accumulates. Yet, our bodies have a simply incredible capacity to rebound and thrive under the right conditions—the conditions created by wellness practice. None of us who believe in self-responsibility for health opts for a long, desolate ride on the Conveyor Belt to a Living Hell. The wellness alternative is just so much more attractive (and so much less expensive in the long run).

There's no denying that life is often tough, demanding an ongoing balancing act to reach fulfillment in all areas we consider important. Wellness helps—a whole lot! Its favorite traveling companions are confidence, vitality, and life-enriching discipline.

I've had my share of ups and downs, like most, and have suffered losses. What has always kept my spirits high is the realization that I have the capacity to remain healthy and fit, and I enjoy the natural support that health and fitness provide. Most importantly, this natural support continues to help me overcome stress—even grief at times—brought on by day-to-day life trials. Knowing what I do about wellness, my health isn't for sale at any price. I consider it my most valuable physical asset. And you?

I've been blessed through the years with a beautiful wife, two wonderful children, loving friends and family, great colleagues, and some marvelous relationships with those whom I've supported, both professionally and personally, in their quests for healing and wellness. And it's these true blessings that make me realize how important it is to maintain my health to the best of my ability. In fact, I consider it irresponsible not to do so. If I don't give my health the priority it deserves, how am I going to properly care for my family? Do I want to risk losing a job and being unable to provide for those who depend on me? Do I want to curtail activity with my children? Do I want to become a burden to those who love me most? I don't accept those risks, and I don't think you want to accept them either if you have a choice. *With rare exceptions, poor health comes from accepting poor information and adopting poor habits.*

What I've discovered about maximum wellness works for me. But it will also work for you and just about anyone who chooses to pursue it. Even so, less committed people will look at your achievements and believe they came from luck or from being genetically gifted when in fact they came mostly from effort, good choices, and good habits.

The truth is this: Few people even begin to approach and hold the level of wellness for which they are capable. Few get even close to achieving the appearance or body shape that's within their grasp—sometimes because they don't want to make the effort, but just as often because they don't know how.

If you're confused about what it takes to achieve maximum wellness and a physical appearance you can be proud of, I can help. If you're looking for a better diet and fitness program than you've followed in the past—or at least tried to follow—I can help. But before explaining how and why I can help you, I first want to make it clear what we're up against when we opt for maximum wellness. Also, why so many people fail to get what they're striving for:

The number one reason most people fail to achieve their wellness goals or even maintain their current state of health is that 90% of the information available to them is inaccurate, distorted, or deliberately misleading.

Does that 90% number seem far-fetched? I can't say that I blame you for thinking so. Actually, I think the number is even higher, but I'm feeling conservative right now! In any event, the credibility of that number will grow on you as you continue to read further. In the chapters that follow, I address this bad-information problem in spades. It has just so many stress-affecting attributes!

So where do we start? First, as a wellness-oriented health practitioner, I consider physical appearance to be one aspect of wellness. The reason is simple: When you look good to yourself and others, your emotional outlook improves, as does your confidence in almost everything you do. Strange how that works, but just think back. Almost surely there were certain periods in your life when your appearance pleased you more than ever and you felt good about it. You were closer to your full physical potential at those times and it showed in different ways. Further, the positive comments that came from others concerning your appearance just added to your sense of pride, confidence, and feeling of well-being, did they not? A positive experience all around.

So, making the effort to attain your best physical appearance is a great catalyst for building your overall health. Although physical appearance is far from being everything, it creates a good foundation. This means attention to your body shape and tone definitely should be a part of your program unless you just can't handle it physically. I'll show you the most efficient and effective ways to do this, based on plenty of up-to-date research. I'll also tell you why the most common approaches don't work so well, or why they won't fit your busy lifestyle.

Actually, my interest in the human physique emerged when I was 12 years old. I was reading about "Mr. America" and was impressed with his appearance when compared to the average guy on the street. But something else also caught my attention: how he carried himself. From that point on, I began to notice that the men and women who kept themselves in the best shape seemed to have an air about them—as if they held some secret. Others certainly admired their appearance and the energy they seemed to bring to life. Was this just coincidence, or did the overall outlook and confidence of these fitness advocates stem from maintaining their health and bodies?

Now, after 30 years of dedicating myself in different ways to understanding and practicing the rituals of caring for one's health, I can confidently say that the people I admired in my younger years knew something that the public didn't:

The presence of optimal health provides for the enjoyment of a richer life—a life that includes family, friendships, career, and any interests or avocations that make you who you are. Moreover, the optimal health or maximum wellness maintained through consistent practice gives you a layer of protection during hard times.

Please note the key word *practice*. To practice doesn't mean to talk about or hope for. As a wellness specialist with a chiropractic background, I've examined thousands of patients suffering from musculoskeletal and general health complaints. As a rule, the patients who take the least care of themselves over the years suffer the most complaints. Accompanying the primary musculoskeletal symptoms are stories of fatigue, loss of energy, intermittent depression, weight gain, and a general loss of youthful vitality. What's happening here?

Well, you already know the answer. If people don't properly care for themselves—if they don't get into the habit of *practicing* optimal wellness—they likely end up taking a long ride on that Conveyor Belt to a Living Hell. And make no mistake about it: achieving and maintaining optimal health takes practice, just as a professional musician must practice daily to stay in top form. Oh, yes, a tiny percentage of genetically anomalous people seem to enjoy optimal health with little or no practice, at least for a time. Well, I don't fit that profile. It's a safe bet you don't, either.

Actually, most people do care about their health. At one time or another, they've attempted to lose weight or tone up with some form of exercise, diet, or both. So why do the majority of hopefuls give up within a month and stash their barely used fitness equipment in the garage, attic, or under their beds? Because the information they've received regarding exercise and diet is wrong, wrong, wrong, and this wrong information messes up their efforts at practicing maximum wellness. They easily lose the passion they had at the outset.

For the next few moments, please picture yourself as lead character in the following fitness drama:

The Fitness Seeker's Lament

You resolve to get in shape, and this time you have an intelligent purpose, an action plan, and a gush of passion to carry through with it. You visit the gym as often as you can, sometimes when you don't feel like it. You even change your diet so fast food is no longer your meal of choice. After six weeks you check yourself. Results? Negligible.

Okay, not being one to give up easily, you continue for another 6 or even 10 weeks, only to discover you've lost but a few pounds, and a few body parts are a little firmer. Well, great—except that with all the lifestyle changes you've made and discipline you've had to conjure up, you should have seen dramatic changes by this time.

You tell your friends about your efforts, fishing for a little validation. They squint at you, looking for the changes you hope they can see. You challenge them to touch or squeeze a G- or PG-rated body part that you claim has yielded to your discipline. They humor you as they squeeze, not wishing to alienate you as a friend.

So tell me—by the end of the above imaginary scenario, what are the chances you still have the same motivation that fired you up at the outset? What happened to that gush of passion that propelled you forward?

Once again, that was just an imaginary scenario, right? No connection with your real-life experience.

So, what have you been doing wrong? Here are some possibilities.

- You've been looking for your inspiration in all the wrong places. The people, organizations, or knowledge sources you have trusted to give you good information may not deserve your trust!

- You *know* you've been following poor fitness habits, but you don't know the best ways to turn that around.
- You've been mesmerized by the sale of junk fitness equipment.
- Your fitness programs haven't fit your lifestyle.
- You've been spending too much time with your fitness training and may actually be harming yourself.
- You haven't chosen a program intended to keep you fit for life!
- You carry a lot of hope about how you'd like life to turn out for you, but you don't contribute much otherwise. Hope is not an action plan!
- You're not using common sense! For example, if you are getting fitness information from someone, how do *they* look? That's the real test. How long have they looked that way? If they look good, do they lead a balanced life of wellness in all its dimensions, or do they spend most of their spare time in a gym carrying on as a one-dimensional creature?

* * *

When you get the *correct* information, and you understand and use it, you *will* succeed. The key is that *the correct information must be at the foundation of your program*. If it isn't, your chances for long-term success diminish greatly, even if you start out with purpose, plan, and passion. Through many years of research in the fields of resistance training, nutrition, approaches to wellness, and the physiology of muscle hypertrophy (an increase in muscle size and density), I've learned about the myths that destroy health and fitness programs. But I've also learned about the secrets to increasing one's chances for a richer life. And if you read the rest of this book, you'll learn what I've learned—only a whole lot easier!

Now, let's revisit those three magic phrases: purpose, action plan, and the passion to proceed. They are, in truth, the three anchors of success in the physical side of your wellness practice—*so long as you build your foundation with the right information!* Plant those anchors in soft ground (the wrong information) and your program will topple with the slightest tremor. Here's how these three anchors of success support your maximum wellness efforts:

❑ You need a compelling *purpose* to act, one to propel you in the right direction and motivate you to undertake a plan designed to get you what you want.

❑ You need a sound *action plan* so you have something concrete to work with and strive for, right from day one—a plan that brings some *quick, significant results* to show you that you're indeed on the right track.

❑ You need a *passion* for wellness that not only fires your imagination so you can see what a future with maximum wellness looks like, but a passion that inspires you to warmly embrace the continued discipline needed to carry through with your *action plan.*

Does that make sense?

Reclaim 24 is a powerful challenge for us to take back the wellness, youth, and vibrancy that we may have allowed to slip through our fingers through self-neglect or through ignorance of the anti-aging "secrets" that I reveal in this book. And just what makes these anti-aging secrets so secret? Well, I want to be straight with you because I'm not crazy about marketing hype. It's not so much that everything has intentionally been hidden from us (though at times it is and has been), but it takes oh so darn long for old myths to die! The truth often hides in the shadows of myths for decades or more.

Most people, including many doctors and other health professionals, just won't let go of the myths. Or they are unable to keep up with the rapid changes in the fields of health and wellness. One example is keeping up with the latest scientific findings on permanent, healthful weight loss. But I make it my business to keep up so I can pass these "secrets" on to my patients and others seeking maximum

> *I have been a patient of Dr. Webb's for about four months now and all I can say is WOW. The ability to regain my health to almost 100% has been great.*
>
> *The last time I weighed myself I am 185 and have lost 23 pounds and 10 pant sizes.*
>
> *It is a lifestyle change for the better. I forgot to mention that I do not take high blood pressure, cholesterol or my ulcer medicines anymore. All of these situations have disappeared since I have been on this program.*
>
> *I am the healthiest I have been in 15 years and I am the strongest I have been since two years out of High School. I am 48 years old and looking mighty lean, my friends, family and co-workers cannot believe the change in such a short time.*
>
> *Mark Wayne Henke*
> *San Antonio, TX*

wellness for a fulfilling, vital life that prevails right to the very end.

There is no reason why your 20's should be your peak years. There's no overwhelming reason why you can't "flatten" that peak into a plateau over three, four, five, or even more decades. But in order to live that way, you must stop practicing the mistakes that prevent ageless living—repeated mistakes that eventually make damage recovery and rejuvenation impossible. If we insist on making the same old mistakes, our lives start revolving around drugs, surgery, dependence on medical intervention, and a long, disheartening trip on the Conveyor Belt to a Living Hell. On the other hand, those who practice an inspired program of optimized living dramatically increase their chances of extending their youth and quality of life far beyond what medicine terms "normal."

Part I of this book talks about crystallizing your purpose, a prerequisite for taking smart, decisive action. Part II outlines the 12-week Action Plan for *Reclaim 24* (the proof-of-concept phase of your *Reclaim 24* lifestyle conversion). Part III talks about developing an even greater passion for wellness once you have convinced yourself that the *Reclaim 24* lifestyle is in your best interests. Plant these three anchors into a solid foundation of correct information, and you have a winner! Without all three anchors firmly planted, your program topples.

I've designed the 12-week *Reclaim 24* Action Plan for anyone at any age, regardless of individual fitness expectations. Much of the plan involves tailoring the program to your personal goals, situations, and needs. This program, including its common-sense nutritional approach, allows you to reach your most obvious fitness goals within a reasonable timeframe—as little as 12 weeks. Plus, you feel better and recognize a step-up in your health.

If your goals are even more far-reaching, my program lets you prove conclusively to yourself that you've chosen a remarkable approach that will work for you well into your advancing years. All this without having to turn your life upside down with countless hours at the gym, and without having to adopt ascetic practices that destroy your joy of life. Embrace *good* information—that's the key, along with the three anchors. But to best understand and set the right goals for yourself, you need to look under the hood.

* * *

If your goal is to reach and maintain your full physical potential, my *Reclaim 24* Workout requires that you spend only about two—2—hours a week in fitness training. If your goal is more modest—to simply drop a couple of sizes and maintain that change without changing your current lifestyle very much—you may need to spend as little as 20 to 30 minutes a couple of times each week. I know of few people who can't afford such a small amount of time.

As a practical matter, after 12 weeks of this program, you gain the confidence and experience to make it a permanent part of your life without ever feeling you are depriving yourself of anything. Indeed, my program is designed to help you *practice* wellness and to make fitness part of your lifestyle—from now on. You also come to realize that what you may have originally felt to be sacrifices are not sacrifices at all. So, it's fair to think of the *Reclaim 24* Action Plan not only as your "proof of concept" but also as your springboard—your transition—into practicing a lifetime of wellness. This is the metamorphosis!

Of course, you need to use common sense when starting any fitness program. This has become a cliché, but it's still rock-solid advice: If you feel you may have a health condition that could be aggravated by strenuous exercise, please consult your doctor before starting. It could save you lots of grief! I certainly would want my patients to do that. It's important to begin slowly and learn the basics as well as your limits. Within a week or two, you are well on your way. Most of all, you are enjoying this program and the lifelong benefits that accompany it.

Let's now shift to the next chapter and take a better look at "wellness" and what it means with respect to your metamorphosis and the *Reclaim 24* lifestyle. Right now, the word "wellness" is largely a buzzword for most people—a stock phrase with a lot of touchy-feely sentiment. But it's also fuzzy in common usage. I think we can do better than that. I want to tie "wellness" down for you so that you can better evaluate the copious information supposedly dedicated to health and wellbeing that flows to and around you every day, much of it erroneous. You, a potential self-care practitioner, need to become a levelheaded consumer of healthy lifestyle information!

More *Reclaim 24* Experiences ...

"At Dr. Webb's, I have made significant progress in healing from long-term acid reflux, and have reduced the use of reflux medications by over 50% and still reducing. I have better digestion, less fatigue and neck pain is much improved. I have also gained so much knowledge about how to be pro-active about my family's health.

"The enthusiasm and warmth of the entire staff and docs for my family's health and wellness is impressive.

"I certainly have and would recommend family and friends to Dr. Webb's Imagine Wellness Centre because there is a wealth of knowledge here that can be used to get to the root of any health problem and resolve most in a healthier manner rather than just masking it with a pill and triggering another health problem with a side effect down the road."

Doretta, Max and Quin Hudler
At-home mom and homeschooler
San Antonio, TX

"Between my first exam with Dr. Webb and the first re-exam, I lost 10 lbs. Wow! My jeans literally fall off now without a belt and I feel great. I'm impressed by how efficient the office visits are – I get in and out. Yet, everything is very thorough from the scans and exams, to the nutrition and workout program.

"I have learned to eat properly and actually enjoy it and I feel great. As a result, my wife and I have been talking to friends and family about Dr. Webb's program."

Reid Fitzgerald
Sales-Telecom
San Antonio, TX

2: Introduction to the Wellness Paradigm

"Whatever you can do, or dream you can do, begin it.
Boldness has genius, power and magic in it. Begin it now."

– Goethe

"The best time to plant a tree was 20 years ago.
The next best time is today."

– Chinese Proverb

Be honest. Do you like what you see when you look in the mirror—especially a full-length mirror? Do you want to turn back the hands of time? Has your quality of life been diminishing a little here and a little there because the appearance, health, energy, and resilience you took for granted in your younger years are slowly slipping from your grasp? Then you are experiencing the first crucial incentive for adopting a wellness lifestyle: *You do not like what is happening to you physically.*

Perhaps you've already tried to do something about it but feel stymied because you don't know what steps to take next. It's easy to be boggled by the conflicting lifestyle advice of family, friends, and countless "authorities" on the subject. Hundreds of approaches, programs, systems, and fads are pitched as the best ways to develop health and fitness. To further complicate matters, the modern push toward wellness is only a few decades old and is still trying to find its place in the hearts and minds of a medicine-and-drug-oriented American public. This is a public addicted to quick fixes. It is a public dependent on doctors and hope to deliver sick individuals from the misery of poor choices and bad habits.

Health and fitness systems flood the infomercials and fill millions of pages in books, magazines, newspapers, and now the Internet. Many of these systems or approaches are contradictory, incompatible, or based on myth or misconception. They tug at you from every angle. To make matters worse, many of these supposed health-and-fitness-building systems actually cause harm to those who follow the systems. Some systems even making folks age more quickly!

So, how do you sort all this out and still retain your sanity? How do you tell the difference between myth, fad, and solid advice? How do you know what fits *you* best? To put it succinctly, how in the midst of so

13

much confusion do you reclaim the health, fitness, and vibrancy that have slowly slipped from your grasp over the years?

What Is Wellness?

For those who really like to sink their teeth into the principles of optimized living, I want to bring some clarity to the topic of wellness. From any angle, I'm a wellness doctor. It's important to me that my patients and others whom I advise understand their goals and achievements. I try to make things as clear and as simple as possible. That's one of the hallmarks of my *Reclaim 24* rejuvenation and anti-aging lifestyle system. I do it by cutting out wasted effort, debunking harmful myths, and exposing the propaganda of Big Pharma and the processed food industry ("fake foods industry" is probably a more fitting phrase). The result is a streamlined approach for optimizing your quality of life, an approach you can live with.

"Wellness" is quite the buzzword these days. To most people, even supposed "authorities," its meaning is fuzzy, abstract, or both—as I'll show you in this chapter. That's understandable. Wellness practice is evolving rapidly and is not so easy to keep up with. One indication of this fuzziness is that the terms "health" and "wellness" are often confused or used interchangeably. Ask a bunch of people, including wellness experts, to cite the difference between health and wellness and you'll see why.

For further entertainment and variety, Google the question, "What is the difference between health and wellness?" Or "What is the difference between health and fitness?" Ideas run the gamut. You'll find little consensus. Though I have opinions to offer that I think can help you wade through the semantic marshes, I'm not about to sort out the semantics for all of humanity! As the public's wellness consciousness continues to rise over the next decade or two, "natural selection" will eventually take care of the fuzziness and abstraction of word usage.

Yet, despite the fuzziness and abstraction, we can still get our arms around some important points. *Wellness* and *wellness practice* represent a new paradigm that really didn't become popular until the 1970's in this country. The wellness mindset differs markedly from the conventional sickness mindset, which requires battling disease to achieve health. The main theme behind sickness practice says that if you have no disease or signs of disease such as high blood pressure, and if you feel pretty good, then you have health. In other words, by convention, health equals freedom from disease and disease symptoms.

But *wellness practice raises the bar much higher than that.* It defines and achieves health differently. It exhibits a holistic mindset that considers optimized living to be a wide-spectrum, multi-dimensional approach that continues to expand over an individual's lifetime. Most important, those who have been dipping their toes into wellness waters are reporting enormous gratification.

Adopting a Passion for Wellness, Part III of this book, goes into the wellness topic in much greater detail. I think you'll be impressed about how much we've been learning since the 1970's about this abstract thing called wellness.

What are some contemporary thoughts on wellness? The website at www.mybindi.com cited four quotations that provide good insight. I'll reproduce them here as contemporary samples and add my assessments:

Sample 1: The online Merriam-Webster dictionary defines wellness as, *"The quality or state of being in good health especially as an actively sought goal."* This is a rudimentary definition that makes some people happy. It's pretty limited, though.

Sample 2: The National Wellness Institute defines wellness as *"... an active process of becoming aware of and making choices toward a more successful existence."* Since moving toward a "more successful existence" seems to encompass more than the "state being in good health," this makes greater sense to me than Sample 1. Further, since "becoming aware" and "making choices toward a more successful existence" is a never-ending process, we can see that this sample implies growth in consciousness. And it hints that there is no endpoint. Nonetheless, this definition seems to confuse *wellness* with *wellness practice,* whereas the first sample doesn't (it just defines wellness).

Sample 3: The Arizona State University definition is similar to the Wellness Institute definition, but is more comprehensive: *"Wellness is an active, lifelong process of becoming aware of choices and making decisions toward a more balanced and fulfilling life. Wellness involves choices about our lives and our priorities that determine our lifestyles."* To me, this is a good definition of *wellness practice*: becoming aware of choices, setting lifestyle priorities, and making decisions that lead to a balanced and fulfilling life. It doesn't make for a good definition of wellness, however. Wellness is like happiness. Happiness isn't a process, it's a desirable state of being!

Sample 4: Economist Paul Zane Pilzer says wellness is *"not a fad or trend, it's about a new and infinite need infusing itself into the way we eat, exercise, sleep, work, save, age, and almost every other aspect of our lives... The sickness business is reactive... The wellness business is proactive."* This is good insight into the wellness practice, but doesn't serve so well as a definition of wellness.

So, there you have a sample of credible *ideas* about wellness, but they just serve to show that the topic is far from concrete in the collective mind.

It's safe to say that health in the 21st century is much more than freedom from disease. And it's more than "feeling good." It's also safe to say that the idea of wellness is incredibly comprehensive and not at all simple to describe if we consider the range of definitions or understandings listed above. Yet, each of the four viewpoints has merit we can build upon for our benefit.

Can we extract a common denominator from those contemporary views of wellness? A common denominator that leaves us with a *working* definition of wellness, a strong feeling for the wellness principle that doesn't require so many mental gyrations? Yes, there is, and it has to do with stress.

Knowing what I do about stress and its wide-ranging effects on our lives and well-being, it makes great sense to relate the idea of wellness to stress, a concept with which we all have gut-level familiarity. After all, stress is the common thread or theme in our lives that justifies the idea of wellness practice in the first place. So, this is how I define wellness in the context of a *Reclaim 24* lifestyle:

> *Wellness* **is the heightened ability to protect ourselves from the physical, emotional, and mental effects of stress.**

See how that fits? Wellness is an overall state of protective conditioning against stress that reaches beyond the ordinary, the mundane. And a *Reclaim 24* lifestyle definitely reaches beyond the ordinary.

Okay. If we're going to define "wellness" as I just did, then it becomes much easier to define "wellness practice" because it springs directly from what we are trying to achieve with wellness. It follows that:

> *Wellness practice* is the adoption of long-term, personal lifestyle behaviors that minimize the onset and impact of unwanted physical, emotional, and mental stress.

This means that when we *practice* wellness, we are recognizing the presence of stress, where it comes from, its positive and negative attributes, and how we can best manage it so it doesn't turn into *dis*tress and diminish our quality of life. *This is the practice of optimized living.*

There is much to learn. A *Reclaim 24* lifestyle has you continually discovering how to manage stress on a day-to-day and moment-to-moment basis. And it is a practical lifestyle. Furthermore, Part III of this book raises the idea of wellness practice to a level that few health advocates have taken it—not because they can't get there, but because it's so hard to find the best information on how to do it. That information was spread all around until I wrote this book and compiled it.

Wellness Isn't for Sheep

It takes effort to practice wellness. You need an inspiring purpose, an action plan, and a life-long passion to make wellness your own. Why? *Because the practice of maximum wellness is 95% self-care!* The remaining 5% is for professional care and consultation.

I often use terms like "maximum wellness," or "optimized wellness," or even "optimized living." There's a reason for that. Each of us is different in the degree to which we can achieve wellness because of many life factors. For example, our history of stress buildup, injury, or handicap plays a large role in how we measure progress along our personal wellness paths. Genetics also plays a role—much less than most people think. And so do attitudes and life situations. So your maximum wellness and my maximum wellness are apt to be different.

In other words, many variables are present that affect each individual, including the degree to which we have educated ourselves about wellness. So, it's silly to think there is some measurable, fixed level of wellness to which everyone should aspire, or some scale along which one can measure it. There isn't. Of course, there are many excellent physiological and psychological tests of well-being that doctors can use to assess where effort should be placed or how one might achieve a better balance or response to stress. However, you'll never hear any reputable doctor report that your wellness level is 47 and that you'll need to get it up to 53 or your love life will fall apart. As you'll learn, wellness has too many dimensions to assign a single number to it reliably!

Therefore, the outward expression of wellness varies across individuals. Yet, what *you* can do is to aspire to the maximum wellness level that life and nature permit *you* to achieve if you dedicate yourself to good self-care plus interaction with wellness professionals. That's what I want *Reclaim 24* to do for you. You don't have to settle for a "little bit of wellness." Or 50% of your personal wellness potential. Or 80%. I urge you not to settle for halfway measures because you only get halfway results. The neat thing about wellness practice is that you can continually step it up as you learn more about what it is and what it can do for you. From this comes the health and optimized living you desire.

At the time I decided to write this book, I had a dream of reaching people who sincerely wanted to reclaim their vitality but were weary of the same old hype and bogus information about wellness, especially the physical appearance and body-shaping aspects. I knew I could help them change old, ingrained thought patterns that would make a dramatic difference in their lives and the lives of those they touch.

You're obviously concerned about your health and appearance, as otherwise you wouldn't still be reading. *Fitness, health, wellness*—each of these has its own shade of meaning and involves a certain motivation that must be understood by anyone who wants to get the most out of this lifetime. As you read on, you'll now see more clearly how these pieces fit together with respect to stress and stress management.

* * *

"Stress equals aging. Reduce stress in all its forms, and aging suddenly slows—dramatically. This is a message that Dr. Webb carries with him at all times. But he also shows you how to do it with his Reclaim 24 approach for quickly reclaiming health, youth, and quality of life through youth-preserving habits. This is important work!"

Loral Langemeier
National Bestseller Author, Mentor
"The Millionaire Maker"

3: Meeting Stress with Open Eyes

It actually starts when you are in your teens and early twenties, but you don't notice it. *Yet it keeps on building*. Then one morning when you least expect it, you look into the mirror, wonder who you're looking at, and in your head hear yourself saying,

"Where is my quality of life going? I don't want to grow old, sick and fat!"

This leads to a kind of depression that simply ruins your day—and maybe many days to follow. You're thinking that age has caught up with you and you're not sure what to do next. And maybe you're thinking that birthday celebrations are not as welcome as they once were. If you resign yourself to accept, at face value, the deterioration you see and feel—if you grow depressed and passive as most people do at this juncture—can grunts, groans, and whimpers be far behind?

Here's the crux of the matter. It's not really calendar age that is stealing your quality of life. If you think about it, the flow of time—if such a thing even exists—is but a *record* of changes. Believing that time is your enemy leads to all sorts of errors in thinking and bad wellness choices. So, what is really causing the unwelcome changes you see in yourself if it's not time?

Built-up damage from stress.

That's right. It's not the passage of calendar years that creates the symptoms of "aging" and deterioration that we see and feel. Rather, what gets to us is stress that we don't have the health to handle as it comes. Therefore, it just "piles up" in the form of negative conditions that we experience physically, mentally, and emotionally.

It's true that no one can escape stress or its buildup. Life and nature pretty much dictate external conditions for the most part, but here's the secret as I see it:

> **Unlike the passage of time, the *rate* of stress buildup—a buildup that eventually leads to our physical demise—is very much under our control!**

No, you can't change your calendar age, but you can resist or even reverse years of stress damage if you're not too late and if not too much damage has already been done. You may have to pay the price for growing up with poor health and wellness choices and for continuing to make them. Yet, you can reverse *much* of the damage because of natural healing abilities that you unleash when you start to make better, more-informed choices. The sooner you start, the better the results. It's all about learning science-based secrets for "ageless" living and shattering the perpetual health myths that cloud the vision of so many of us. With this approach—the advanced *Reclaim 24* approach—you are able to get a handle on runaway stress and its effects. With this comes the start of optimized living.

Early Hints of Runaway Stress

We get plenty of forewarning about runaway stress—from many directions. Here are common signs of runaway stress. Even if you haven't experienced some of them yourself, I'm sure they won't surprise you. But if you are interested in optimized living, you must be able to recognize runaway stress when you see it (or feel it):

- You cringe in front of a mirror because of growing rolls of fat, fading muscle tone, or unmistakable signs of "premature aging."
- Aches, pains, and a foggy brain have become your closest friends.
- You *feel* tension. You're irritable. You aren't able to concentrate.
- You experience dry mouth, teeth grinding, sweaty palms or cold hands, a pounding heart, shallow breathing, chronic headache, low self-esteem, or withdrawal.
- Your sleep quality is in the pits, and exhaustion rules your day.
- You get an upset stomach or urinate frequently.
- You have a lowered sex drive. (Note: even if you prefer "not to be bothered," a low sex drive and is always a sign that something else is wrong behind the scenes. It also puts "stress" on relationships.)
- Your workouts are, well, not working out!
- You have nervous twitches or tight muscles that cause pain and trembling.

- You sense your hormone balances are all out of whack, but you have no idea what to do about it other than suffer.

- Your single greatest weapon for warding off surgery or chronic disease is hope.

- You are handling your quality-of-life problems with stimulants, products from a drugstore, and/or the services of "sickness care" professionals.

- Your medical doctor has you worried about the "numbers" from your last physical exam; and daily, stress-building medications could soon become part of your lifestyle if they haven't already.

- As a spouse, parent, lover, friend, business owner, employee, student, fitness seeker, or creative worker, your *lackluster performance* is leaving others out in the cold—and you're not feeling very warm about it, either!

Got stress?

Placing Stress under a Microscope

Okay. Since the *Reclaim 24* lifestyle places so much emphasis on understanding and managing stress, this is a good time to get our arms around it. However, you won't have to commit this "microscope" section to memory to practice wellness successfully. It's intended for those who like details.

In common use, the word "stress" covers a lot of ground. It carries at least three, closely related yet different meanings, depending on the context. See if the meanings make sense to you in your experience:

1. Stress sometimes means a collection of things that are happening in your life to throw you out of a "normal" state of balance or security. It constitutes those situations or conditions that pull you out of your physical, mental, and emotional comfort zones—or even threaten your survival. In formal language, these "things" are called "stressors." Examples of stressors are worry, repetitive motions, fear in dangerous situations, job loss, **strength training, the excitement of riding a roller coaster, getting a job promotion, or falling in love.** Please note that the first four examples are what we usually think of as negative stress or "distress," while the last four are examples of positive stress, or

"eustress" (see the sidebar) The important thing to remember is that when stressors touch our lives, the body cannot recognize the difference between distress and eustress. It responds in the same, *automatic* ways—as in #2.

2. In common usage stress also means your body's automatic *reactions* to your being pulled out of your physical, mental, and emotional comfort zones. This type of stress is the closest to your conscious awareness and closest to the classical definition in Hans Seyle's original book, *Stress and Distress* (Seyle was the founder of stress theory).

   This is the stress you can often feel. Here, your body is calling on its chemical and energy "reserves" to deal with both distress and eustress. These reactions are your body's physiological protectors. If you have enough reserves, you get along quite well. *Those who practice wellness have more reserves than those who don't.*

   > *Eustress* is actually important for us to have in our lives. It keeps us vital and excited. Without it, we would become depressed and perhaps feel a lack of meaning in life. Not striving for goals, not overcoming challenges, not having a reason to wake up in the morning would be damaging to us, so eustress is considered 'good' stress. It keeps us healthy and happy.
   > – about.com

3. Finally, stress is sometimes taken to mean your body's innate *compensation* for dealing with those situations where the reserves of #2 simply fall short. Here we're talking about what happens to the body when the reserves of #2 are simply not enough, either because they have been depleted from earlier attempts at rebalance, or because the stress load is just too large to handle, even for someone with good reserves. That's why some call this condition *overstress*.

   Overstress can and does "build up" and lead to things such as insomnia, exhaustion, premature aging, weight gain, and many more conditions too numerous to mention. If unattended, stress buildup can seriously damage physical health, psychological well-being, and relationships with friends, family, and coworkers. When it builds enough, the results are disease, infirmity, or even death.

In reality, death is the body's final compensation for stress buildup. Stress has won, as it always does, because that's nature's way. But those with high wellness I.Q.s don't throw in the towel early. They find that life is much too valuable to be spending years or even decades mired in illness or feeling poorly (riding the Conveyor Belt to a Living Hell). And they know they have a choice through intelligent self-care.

So, to put these three shades of "stress" into perspective, it goes something like this: With meaning #1, you might say, "There's a lot of stress at my workplace." With meaning #2, "I feel stressed when I'm at work." And with meaning #3, "I'm stressed from too much work and need to take a vacation so I can recuperate." It's sometimes good to notice these shades of common usage although they usually won't cause too much confusion in conversation. People catch the drift (or at least they think they do).

Your Body's Automatic Stress-Protection System

In the physiological sense, stress (type #2) is your body's *automatic* attempt to protect itself from injury or perceived dangers, *whether real or imagined*. When such "dangers" loom, your body's reactions include the following signs and symptoms, commonly called the *fight or flight response:*

- Increased secretion of adrenalin.
- Elevated blood pressure.
- Accelerated heartbeat.
- Greater muscle tension.
- A slowed or halted digestion.
- A release of fats and sugars from body stores.
- An elevation of cholesterol levels.
- A slight change in blood composition, making it more prone to clotting.
- An increase in the pituitary gland's production of the hormone, ACTH. This in turn stimulates the release of cortisone and cortisol. These inhibit disease-fighting white blood cells and suppress the immune response.

All these bodily reactions occur in the name of protection! And they work just fine for those short-term situations where a heightened ability to react is important for protection and survival. The funny thing is that, today, few of the dangers that our bodies react to result from immediate physical threats or challenges, such as a tiger leaping at us from the underbrush. They come mostly from "modern" physical, chemical, and emotional stressors. Yet, the body still responds with its natural, primitive, "fight or flight" behavior.

Today, hormones and other chemical messengers can pour into a stressed person over many hours of the day and night. Often such individuals have been following lifestyles that attract or inadvertently welcome many threats and dangers, both real and imagined. But the chemicals are not serving their intended short-term, protective purposes. It's hard on a body to be expecting a tiger to jump out of the underbrush many hours a day (for some it's 24/7). The continuous flow of chemicals starts to damage the system rather than protect it. Moreover, the chemicals may simply exhaust themselves so they are no longer available when *really* needed. For example, *adrenal exhaustion* is common in people leading a stressful lifestyle.

When Your Automatic Protection Isn't Enough

Yes, the body tries hard to accommodate modern stressors, but there is only so much it can do. Our protective resources are limited, and we can become overstressed (type #3). The nervous system is one of the first bodily systems to react to the damage.

But there is an upside. In most cases, stress buildup announces itself long before you get into the danger zone. You are in a position to catch it early, before it starts running away with you. If you want to experience the hidden harmonies of optimized living and satisfy your personal wellness potential, you must:

1. Be able to recognize the early symptoms of stress buildup in your body and emotions.
2. Learn how to avoid—or at least sidestep—life challenges that lead to stress buildup.
3. Learn how to heal stress buildup that has already occurred.

And what are some *early* hints of runaway stress? I listed them on page 20.

You can avoid major problems if you identify symptoms of stress early. No, you can't avoid all of life's challenges, and you don't want to avoid all of them because eustress adds richness to life. But the wellness-

24

damaging challenges that you *can* avoid are much greater in number than you think. These are your opportunities to spare your nervous system! They start with taking *personal responsibility* for challenges under your control. Personal responsibility is a huge part of the wellness lifestyle. In fact, a "person of wellness" distinguishes him or herself from the crowd by the level of personal responsibility he or she is willing to take.

The fact is we create many of our own challenges, most often by unwittingly or carelessly inviting them into our lives. By becoming aware of such challenges, we are taking the first step towards eliminating them as agents of stress buildup. Once you know some of your stress symptoms and are aware of when stress is occurring, you can begin to use stress management strategies to deal with them. Many stress experts even believe that how a person deals with stress may be more important than the number or type of demands he or she faces. For example, although physical stress reactions (type #2) are pretty much automatic and governed by the primitive, genetic "wiring" of our nervous systems, emotional stress reactions have more to do with conscious choices and developed habits. That says a lot.

Next, I want to cover the four crucial categories of wellness. Understanding these categories and acting upon what we learn is truly our greatest ally in shattering pharmaceutical and medical fictions that diminish our quality of life. It gives us a chance to live up to our wellness potentials if we choose self-responsibility.

The Four Crucial Categories of Wellness

Chapter 2 introduced practical, working definitions for both "wellness" and "wellness practice," relating them to something quite familiar to all of us—stress. I'll repeat the working definitions here:

Wellness—the <u>heightened ability</u> to protect ourselves from the physical, emotional, and mental effects of stress.

- - -

Wellness Practice—the adoption of <u>personal lifestyle behaviors</u> that minimize the onset and impact of physical, emotional, and mental stress.

Now I want to follow up on what these personal lifestyle behaviors might be.

Authors often break up the wellness topic into pieces that are easier to digest and relate to. I have found, as a practical matter, that the dominant behaviors of wellness self-care fall into four main categories. These categories are physical, emotional, intellectual, and spiritual.[1] Although other authors and researchers might cite additional categories to support their communication intent, I tend to include those additional categories in the basic four for simplicity because my message isn't complex.

At the heart of it all, wellness practice amounts to the continued development of positive, practical abilities over time—*abilities largely subject to self-assessment.* When we break down these abilities into the four main areas, a concrete picture emerges. Our job then is to understand the *opportunities* available to us in that picture, and to follow through in order to develop the cited abilities as best we can. Then we can legitimately call ourselves wellness practitioners!

> **Physical wellness** is the ability to apply your knowledge, motivation, commitment, behavior, self-management, attitude, and skills toward achieving your personal fitness and health goals. You can maintain physical wellness by applying the knowledge and skills of sound nutrition, exercise, youth-extension strategies, and safety to everyday life. Hobbies can even play a large role! Physical wellness is characterized by high energy and vitality; freedom from or high adaptability to pain, dysfunction, and disability; a strong immune system; a body that feels light, balanced, strong, flexible, and has good aerobic capacity; ability to meet physical challenges; and full capacity of all five senses plus a healthy libido.

> **Emotional wellness** is the ability to meet your emotional needs constructively. It involves a positive attitude and the ability to respond resiliently to emotional states and the flow of every-day life. When you have emotional wellness, you can deal with a variety of situations realistically and learn more about yourself and how the things you do affect your feelings. You take responsibility for your own behavior and respond to challenges as opportunities. Emotional wellness is characterized by self-acceptance and high self-esteem; capacity to identify, express, experience, and accept

---

[1] I've aligned my thinking here with that found in Robert S. Ivker's book, *The Complete Self-Care Guide to Holistic Medicine*, Tarcher/Pubnam, New York, 1999, ISBN 0-87477-986-3, pp. 6-7.

all your feelings, whether painful, joyful, or anything in between; freedom from guilt (replaced by self-responsibility); awareness of the intimate connection between your physical and emotional selves; ability to confront your greatest fears; and maintaining and fulfilling your capacity to play.

Intellectual wellness is having a curiosity and strong desire to learn. You value many experiences, stay stimulated with new ideas, and share your discoveries with others where welcomed or when invited. You respond to challenges and opportunities to grow, make plans, develop strategies, and solve problems. You engage in clear thinking and recall. Further, you think independently, creatively, and critically. Intellectual wellness is characterized by optimism; the capacity for peace of mind and contentment; loving what you do and doing what you love; a sense of humor; financial well-being; and preparing and living your life's vision. It has little to do with high IQ or the ability to debate.

Spiritual wellness is being able to look within and work from your spiritual core on a moment-to-moment basis, allowing the spiritual to influence how you view and serve life. Spiritual wellness is characterized by the absence of fear; the ability to love unconditionally; holding a sense of purpose; the ability to be "present" whenever you choose; Soul awareness and a personal relationship with God or Spirit; trust in your intuition and an openness to change; the desire and willingness to smooth the pathway for others as well as yourself; gratitude for the richness and meaningfulness of life, no matter what experiences it brings (plus, gratitude for life, itself); and creation of a "sacred space" on a regular basis through prayer, meditation, contemplation, walking in nature, observing a Sabbath day, or other rituals that you consider sacred—rituals that help promote the relinquishment of lust, anger, greed, vanity, and attachment to material things, to be replaced by the virtues of discrimination, forgiveness, tolerance, contentment, detachment, and humility.

From the above paragraph, how do your rate yourself with respect to spiritual wellness? Life has sped up so much for most of us that the spiritual often gets placed on the back burner—a burner that is sometimes not even turned on low flame! Here's the thing: Because spiritual wellness so deeply affects physical, emotional, and mental wellness and serves to hold all the pieces together, *life tends to fragment without it.*

Ultimately, true healing occurs on the spiritual plane. Then everything else has to catch up. Therefore, our top priority for life should be something of a spiritual nature.

Personally, I don't even think it's possible to achieve maximum wellness without honoring one's spiritual nature, but some try. To me it's like attempting to live a meaningful and fulfilling life with one arm tied behind your back. Research continues to show that people who attend to their spiritual natures serve as beacons of vitality for both themselves and others (that is, as long as they are not encroaching on another's sanctified living and being space). And they live predictably healthier lives.

I'm in no position to tell anyone how to maintain or grow his or her spiritual nature. That's much too personal, too intimate, and too individual for others to muscle in on without invitation. But what I *can* do is tell you what's at the heart of the spiritual temperament—the golden thread that tends to bind all good things together. It's love—that warm, human affection for those who are close to us, and impersonal good will (charity) for *all* others. Trying to live a rich life without these love factors being present in large measure means traveling uphill most of the time. And trying to find love and self-fulfillment through the exercise of power and control over others is an exercise in futility. I've had my say.

> "How do you keep in step with the spiritual laws—and lessen the wear and tear upon yourself? Simply love."
> – Harold Klemp, *The Language of Soul*

* * *

The approach for practicing and achieving wellness that I advocate in this book starts with a physical fitness and nutritional metamorphosis. This science-based fitness regimen, coupled with proper diet and the right types of exercise, can dramatically improve your appearance with only 24 total hours of exercise effort over 12 weeks. And your friends won't have to humor you or guess whether you've achieved an improvement in appearance.

Of course, this metamorphosis makes you feel much better, too! I start with this approach because it parallels my personal interest in appearance and fitness maintenance. It also plays into my professional expertise as a wellness oriented chiropractor. Because the field of wellness is so comprehensive, another author would likely approach it from a different angle. But no matter what angle is taken, physical fitness and appearance are huge parts of overall wellness. There is no getting around that fact.

So here I am, not at all bashful in saying that I believe *Metamorphosis* is the last lifestyle and fitness book you'll ever need to read. But the book isn't just about physical fitness and body shaping. It's about the full scope of wellness as practiced under the *four wellness categories*. It's about *complete* metamorphosis.

Introducing the Five Pillars of Optimized Health

Through practice and experience, I've been able to identify five key components for the health aspect of optimized living. They have become the hallmarks of the *Reclaim 24* basic lifestyle. In my system, I call them *The Five Pillars of Optimized Health*. They are:

1. Nervous system health, from a structural, stress-release perspective

2. Health of organs and glands, especially from a hormonal perspective

3. Detoxification, to reduce toxic stressors

4. Nutrition

5. Fitness, motion, exercise

I address these five pillars throughout the book and then pull them together in the last chapter so you can see how everything fits. Of course, I start with pillars 4 and 5 so you can prove to yourself that you're not wasting your time. You get quick results to serve as an incentive to go further in your wellness practice.

So, in these pages you will find:

❑ An inspiring purpose

❑ A realistic, short-term action plan that proves to you—within only 12 weeks—that you're on the right track

❑ Plenty of justification and support for developing and holding a lifelong passion for wellness so you can rewrite your life experience (and perhaps the life experiences of your family members and others you love).

Here's the thing. *Reclaim 24* is a rejuvenation and wellness blueprint that unleashes your ability to reclaim and experience the hidden harmonies of optimized living, 24 hours a day. Using this blueprint, you exploit your personal wellness potential by following simple, self-care practices and habit changes. These practices cover the physical, emotional, mental, and spiritual areas of your life.

Are you ready to incorporate some rejuvenation and wellness secrets into your life that won't take more time or resources than you can afford to devote? Then let's take this journey together.

* * *

> *"How many people have the knowledge to legitimately teach quality of life from youth well into our senior years? Not many! But Charles Webb can, and does. It's all about unleashing your personal wellness potential through self-care practices. Dr. Webb tells you how, and with self-evident authority."*
>
> *James Malinchak*
> *The Big Money Entrepreneur™*
> *Co-Author, Chicken Soup for the College Soul*
> *"Two Time College Speaker of the Year"*
> *www.Malinchak.com*

> *"As a busy entrepreneur it was always hard for me to follow a training and proper diet routine. Upon utilizing Dr. Webb's program I have found that it really can't be any easier that what he has created! I have transformed my body and my energy level is through the roof! I love it and can see myself doing this for years to come as now it is just a way of life. I would recommend this to anyone at any age or fitness level. Dr. Webb really knows his stuff!"*
>
> *Robert Elder*
> *Summit Award Realtor of the Year*
> *San Antonio, TX*

PART I:
CRYSTALLIZING YOUR PURPOSE

"Dr. Webb and Dr. Boss mentored me through each phase and by following their guidelines; heartburn and indigestion went away almost immediately, chest pain is gone, I lost over 20 pounds and I now sleep through the night.

"I also noticed other changes I am not so anxious anymore. I turned 50 last year and I noticed my libido wasn't what it used to be and now that's increasing yoo-hoo.

"I look forward to the continued improvements that are yet to come. My many thanks go to Dr. Webb, Dr. Boss, and their wellness team."

Ben Rucka
San Antonio, TX

"For a man that is 60 years old, this has been a life changing experience. I've lost inches and fat around my midsection after only 5 weeks on Dr. Webb's program.

"I am looking better every day, and have an overall feeling of vitality and well-being. My strength and physical shape has also improved greatly. People notice and compliments follow.

"The staff is just the best! I've especially enjoyed their personal greetings, friendliness and sincere caring about me and my progress. The personal interest of Drs. Webb and Boss in seeing me get healthier has impressed me as well.

"Because of these fantastic results in such a short time, I have already recommended Dr. Webb's program to my family and friends."

Bob Crittenden, Consultant,
Construction/Development
San Antonio, TX

4: Deciding to Change

Where we are in life right now, including our misfortunes, is largely based on decisions we made in our past. Sure, it's easy to blame someone else for our hardships because we can, but the truth is that embracing good thoughts and taking good actions tend to bring rewards, while poor thoughts and actions tend to bring misfortune. And among these poor thoughts and actions is the habit of assigning blame to others. But here's the thing: *blame is opportunity lost.*

For example, I once lost a lot of money in a company I had purchased after allowing the company's president to continue to run it. It was a grave mistake since the president's interest was vested in another business rather than my company. As I watched the company crumble, I could have pointed the finger of blame at the president, but I soon realized the circumstances were really a result of my poor judgment and poor preparation. I didn't research properly before buying the company, and I was wrong in retaining uncommitted management. As a result of this experience, I'm now careful with making decisions in all aspects of my life because I understand that my future circumstances are forged by present-day decisions.

I share this because I want you to examine your current circumstances in light of past thoughts, actions, and habits. Your financial situation, career, personal relationships, relationship with God, and fitness are all a result of the past. In order to change your future, you must plant better thoughts, make responsible choices, and take decisive action today.

I'm not suggesting that you currently have a terrible life or even an average one, but I do know all of us wish for an even richer life. This is part of our design. We should always strive to achieve all we can in order to earn and share all the rewards and gifts this life has to offer. Anything less is a waste of precious opportunity. As James Allen says in *As a Man Thinketh*, "Every thought seed sown or allowed to fall into the mind, and to take root there, produces its own, blossoming sooner or later into act, and bearing its own fruitage of opportunity. Good thoughts bear good fruit, bad thoughts bad fruit."

> "The human mind is the greatest force on earth. Our thinking (or lack thereof) will take us to our destiny or cause us to abort our dreams. The greatest limitations we have are not external, but those we self-impose because of the way we think."
> – Christine Caine, *Thin Blue Line*

33

If we are not constantly working to improve ourselves, *we do not remain the same*. Rather, we deteriorate in response to the laws of time. If we're not going forward, we're going backward. Staying the same isn't an option for us, though many live as though they have such an option and fight hard for it. (Hint: It doesn't work.)

So how do we begin to make these changes? How can we guarantee that next year brings more pleasant circumstance and rewards than the last few? The answer is really basic and uncomplicated. Though there are uncommon exceptions, the choices we make in life are based on the avoidance of pain or the gain of pleasure. Sounds primitive, doesn't it? Well, it *is* primitive, and for good reason.

Within our DNA lies a survival program designed to make automatic decisions. For the bulk of human history this program has continued to work perfectly and continues to work today for the most part. With today's luxuries, however, we have come to confuse pleasurable circumstances with pleasurable moments. What do I mean by this?

Often we make decisions for immediate gratification without taking into account the longer-term implications. Since this is a wellness support book, let me give a health related example: Deciding to have a large bowl of ice cream an hour before going to bed isn't based on avoiding pain, but rather on gaining pleasure. Is it okay to make a choice based on pleasure? Of course it is—as long as our choice does not lead to a negative circumstance (or we at least take responsibility and accept the consequences of our poor choices). Let's examine this idea more closely.

The first thing is to define pleasure in terms that are more accurate. Will eating a large bowl of ice cream result in a negative circumstance? Probably not much of a circumstance if you do it only periodically. But if this is a daily habit, you obviously need to rethink it. Therefore, the definition of pleasure must include the idea of long-term happiness and long-term results if we want to launch ourselves into a lifetime of wellness. Many people staunchly avoid connecting their short-term desires for pleasure with tomorrow's negatives (which always seem to show up much sooner than expected).

There you have it! Just take a few moments to think about how long each pleasurable experience is going to last when compared with how long the potential negative repercussion remains once the pleasure is long gone. If you don't already think this way, it may take some getting used to, but it's no more difficult than your current way of thinking and making choices. Here's the thing: If you're unwilling to start thinking about wellness in the long-term, you might just as well stop reading now. I certainly can't help you.

The Pain of Remaining the Same

Pain is a great motivator in decision-making. When the pain of remaining the same becomes heavy—when it begins to outweigh the inconvenience or drudgery of developing new habits—that's when we move into action. **In fact, according to research, pain is a stronger motivator to action than pleasure.** You've been there, and more than once. When our job is unbearable, we eventually change employers or even careers, which usually softens the pain and leads to new and better things. When we feel out of shape to the point we've become sick of ourselves, we begin making better choices. This may mean simply going for a walk instead of watching the newest reality show on TV.

Over time, one good decision per day leads to two, then three, and so on until your circumstances change. This does not have to be difficult since there is no race. On the other hand, you need to do enough to make recognizable progress—so that you know when you're putting in enough effort to make a difference. You won't need to have anyone else whisper in your ear to validate your effort. You will know.

If your past actions toward change didn't pan out, your actions may have been faulty. I don't mean your efforts were unworthy. I just mean your actions may have been based on improper information. When it comes to your fitness and wellness, I can assure you the actions I've outlined in this book **will** bring about change and pleasurable circumstances. When your actions make a positive difference, you'll begin to make good decisions consistently.

* * *

"I was tired, worn out, had low energy, and wished that 10 lbs. would just disappear. Did I mention my cholesterol seemed to be going up?

"Now, for the side Effects:

"I sleep all night; enjoy a huge boost in energy and wellbeing; have a great deal more strength; the cholesterol has dropped and so has the weight. I feel good about myself and I am handling the stress of daily life much more effectively."

Janice Schott
Administrative Services
San Antonio, TX

"Before joining the program I wasn't active at all, and now I am very active! I am now able to live a very active lifestyle! My wife is now very happy with my energy level and how interactive I am with her. This is very healthy for our marriage.

"The education and the visits will benefit you long term if you just follow the program. Listen to what they have to say. This is a great solution to any problem that you are having. At least try it. Listen to what they have to say because it does work!!!"

Tim Spellman
HEB Store Director
San Antonio, TX

5: Breaking Old Habits
The Challenges and Rewards

"Thoughts are the threads that bind us to deeds.
Deeds are the ropes that bind us to habits.
Habits are the chains that bind us to destiny."

- Inscription carved on the West Wall at the Palace in Maygassa

Periodically, all of us have had to deal with bad habits. It seems that once we acquire them, they take up shop and move into our subconscious mind on a permanent basis. We know that bad habits lead to no good, yet we continue to allow them to rule over our God-given decision-making abilities. Why is this so? Is it because we are just primitive thinking beasts with no capacity to make thoughtful decisions at all?

Of course not.

We are more than capable of making decisions based on our understanding of the desired outcomes. In other words, if I choose to smoke a pack of Camel cigarettes every day because I enjoy it (pleasure), I know I'm putting my present health as well as my future quality of life at risk (likely deferred pain). Yet, so many Americans make this very decision every day, day after day, knowing that they are throwing the dice and hoping to have their cake and eat it too. But the odds overwhelmingly favor the "The House of Pain and Anguish" (or the Pits of Despair at the end of the Conveyor Belt to a Living Hell).

In the case of cigarettes, evidence has proven smoking is addictive, which of course makes it harder for users to quit. However, the pain associated with quitting is certainly not physical except for an occasional headache; it's mental or psychological. This means the addicted smoker chooses to continue the nicotine habit not to avoid pain, but to gain the short-term, mood-altering pleasure that comes from nicotine.

Habits are formed within the neurological framework of the mind. Just as a stream of running water cuts pathways into the earth, habits shape neuronal paths within the nervous system. Once these paths have formed, it's easier to follow the learned behavior than to change it. The good news is that all habits can be changed the same way they were created … one day at a time. It takes four to six weeks for these neuronal paths to form, and the same amount of time to revise or interrupt them.

Can you take six weeks out of your approximately 4,160 weeks of life to break bad habits? You can if you know how to *replace them* with habits that bring results. Remember, you're more likely to continue something if the outcome brings pleasure. Doubly so if you're simultaneously removing pain.

You must adopt one important behavior if you're to achieve continued success in letting go of nasty habits: DON'T FOCUS ON GETTING RID OF THEM! Why I point this out becomes clearer in the discussion of the subconscious mind. I'm sure you've heard a phrase similar to, "We receive not the things we want or need, but the things we focus on the most." If we focus on love, we have a good chance of receiving it—especially if we understand how the laws of reciprocation work. If we focus on poverty, we are sure to miss our prospects for finding riches. If we focus on the negative aspects of our health, we miss the blessings we have within us to reach our health and fitness **potentials**. And this particular focus is all about *what we choose to be picturing in our imagination.*

Don't make the mistake of thinking bad habits such as smoking, excessive coffee drinking, or frequent sugar infusions are friends or comforting partners in life. They are fickle friends that offer nothing to you except burdens that keep you from fulfilling your dreams. When giving them up, don't imagine yourself losing something. Rather, focus on the fact that you're gaining your freedom (and possibly some extra money in your pocket). Every bad habit that you drop needs to have the void filled again, whether with a good habit or another bad habit. The vacuum <u>must</u> be filled. You make the choice by where you place your attention.

> *"Think of all the things you do today that are nothing more than habits. Good or bad—you formed them through repetition of thought—and repetition of deed.*
>
> *"The truth about the formation of habits is that they start out as ideas—then you act upon them. And if you act upon them every day for 28 days, sometimes less, the habit is locked in. Virtue or vice—the habit has YOU—you don't have it."* – Matt Furey, mattfurey.com

On the other hand, avoid like the plague looking at yourself from afar, as though you don't want to associate with who you currently are. If you would welcome warm friendships with others despite their being out of shape or having some extra blubber on their bones, you must not treat yourself differently. To do so is really quite destructive. The reality is you are who you are at this moment. This is your starting point. And every day is a new starting point. If you wouldn't want others looking down their noses at who you are—right now—don't be doing it to yourself. Instead, just keep focused on the simplicity of what this program is helping you do: detach some bad habits and attach some good ones. From this you get benefits you can enjoy.

So let's say you're now thinking about your negative habits and how you can replace them. The first thing you need to do is make certain your friends and family have a clear understanding that you've chosen to drop some of your common habits. Unfortunately, misery likes company. Your friends and family may not be so enthusiastic about your new choices since your choices may make them feel guilty about their own. Have you ever felt guilty when a close friend of yours stepped up to the plate to make some common-sense changes that you weren't ready or willing to make yourself?

In truth, bad habits are mutually shared amongst friends because we tend to associate with people with similar interests, including some not-so-constructive interests. We are relational beings, and the typical ways we relate are through common interests, hobbies, activities—and habits. The bottom-line question is this: Are you going to allow *your friends'* lack of willpower or interest for changing their lives to affect your decisions about changing *yours*?

At the outset, the impact of friends and family on your efforts at gaining fitness may not seem like such a big deal, but if you've ever tried to step out of your comfort zone, you know it's often friends and family who dampen your enthusiasm the most. They may not want you to change or lose habits you have in common with them because they don't want to let go of their own. Do you want those kinds of friends in your life? Is their companionship worth the price you must pay?

It's truly a sad note about human nature that the average person will try to discourage another's dream that strives to reach beyond the ordinary. This attitude is the great social leveler. It's an attitude that vilifies excellence. Be alert. It's happening all around you.

So, if a goal is important to you, keep quiet about it—or only share it with one or two close, trusted friends. Be sure they have given support to your past dreams and goals. Such encouragement can help.

Now, I'm not suggesting you drop all your friends and start over, but practicalities might require that you step back from those few who do not support your efforts in achieving your fitness or wellness goals. Stepping back from some non-supportive family members might be harder, of course, if not totally unworkable. Life has its burdens. We need to fire up our creative imaginations to handle those burdens.

The Breath of Freedom!

As you start to let go of old, worn-out habits that have kept you stagnant for years, you begin to feel a sense of freedom. It's really quite beautiful to feel that you're actually in control of your future. It's like waking up on a bright, fresh spring morning after a good night's rest with no commitments for the day! When you finally replace those negative habits with positive ones, nothing will keep you from seizing and taking advantage of your wonderful life.

Aside from the obvious health benefits, what else have you been missing by remaining the same? In your mind's eye, take a good look at what you've been missing—since it's going to be one of the goals you're going to move toward. Might it be a positive self-image? With an improved self-image come self-respect and discipline. With self-respect and discipline comes the desire to take on new challenges in life. As you take on new challenges, you gain confidence. Then along with confidence arises the new habit of projecting your positive best for the benefit of others. Positive thoughts and behavior toward family, friends and co-workers lead to others stepping out of their comfort zones and taking control of their lives as well as supporting your efforts. It's amazing how all these benefits accrue and follow on the heels of each other just by starting along a pathway that embraces a positive self-image!

Can Anyone Change?

Do you wonder whether you really have it in you to make the necessary changes? You may have given up years ago and convinced yourself that there are other things in life to focus on besides your health and appearance. You may comfort yourself by saying, "Focusing too much on my appearance is just selfish and is only for those who need to boost their self-confidence. My family and job are my real responsibilities. I don't count enough to take time away from those responsibilities."

Does that sound familiar? If it does, you're simply attempting to convince yourself that it's all right to neglect yourself. Now, whom in this world are you possibly going to benefit by neglecting yourself year after year until your health and emotional state deteriorate? As Zig Ziglar has often said, that is just pure "stinking thinking." Are you just settling into *today's path of least resistance* without thinking of *tomorrow's consequences*? Do you not see how tomorrow's barriers to health and fitness become simply awful, if not insurmountable, if you carelessly sidestep today's opportunities to smooth your pathway into the future?

Okay. If you're like most other people, you consider it a major problem to find the time in your hectic schedule to change your behaviors. Here's a little secret. **Time is always a problem (real or imagined) no matter who you are or what you do for a living!**

Lack of time is the most flimsy of all excuses, but it's the easiest, most convenient one to use. Many people find time to take care of themselves and exercise while working 40 hours per week. Others who work two jobs and 70 hours per week also "find" the time. In truth, there is no time to find. There is only time to allocate. And we allocate based on our chosen priorities. This all boils down to choice, simply choice. Don't fool yourself with the time excuse. You're the one who loses.

I often hear my patients make statements that they would love to get into better shape; however, there just simply isn't enough time in the day. When I ask them to tell me the approximate number of hours of television they watch per week, my question is met with silence.

Have you ever calculated this number for your own curiosity? Did you know the average American spends nearly 30 hours per week glued to his or her screen? The *Reclaim 24* Workout requires *a maximum of two hours per week out of 112 total waking hours.* I said a *maximum* of two hours, which means substantial results can still be achieved in half that amount of time. Now can you honestly convince yourself that you cannot spare $1/50^{th}$ to $1/100^{th}$ of your allocated time toward caring for yourself? A wise person once said, "Those who think they have no time for exercise sooner or later have to find time for illness."

Earlier I made the claim that my health was my most valuable asset. Many well-intentioned people would say mine is a selfish position since my wife and children should be first in my life. But the fact is this: my family *IS* the reason I must make my health my number one asset.

In truth, I find it selfish to languish in deceptively comfortable, old habits that preclude adequately taking care of myself. Such self-abuse ultimately hurts my loved ones. Does this make sense? Deny yourself proper care today, and both you and your family pay the price of neglect tomorrow. But there are many health gamblers out there betting against the House of Pain and Anguish (run by drug companies, negative medical practices, hospitals, and long-term care facilities). In case you haven't noticed, the House is doing very well and welcomes these gamblers with open arms! Follow the money and you'll see what I mean.

Over the past 20 years I've had the opportunity to work with thousands of patients and have seen countless families devastated by serious illnesses and debilitating diseases affecting their spouses, parents, or grandparents. Most of these conditions have been brought on by inactivity and obesity, and therefore can usually be avoided. If you judge yourself a supportive human being and you want to place your loved ones above everything, then you absolutely need to re-think your attitude toward reordering your time priorities and caring for yourself. Remember, your time with the *Reclaim 24* program will be well spent because it induces changes that bring greater joy of life not only to you, but to your family as well. It's the joy of being able to be there, with full personal resources, for those who you love and who depend on you!

And what's another reason to take care of yourself? Renewed health brings renewed energy. This means you soon find that you're accomplishing more work, completing more activities, and catching up on past projects in less time and with less stress. You'll be amazed to find how much you can do in a day when you have enhanced energy and enthusiasm to work with. Just think—this getting into shape thing might actually bring you more leisure time!

If you still question your ability to move into action and make something happen with the time you have, here's a story to consider. Several years ago, one of my dear friends (I'll call him John) was involved in a motorcycle accident. I remember getting a phone call around 2:00 a.m. from a mutual friend telling me the news. His voice betrayed his anxiety as he waited at the hospital to hear the seriousness of John's condition.

When I arrived at the hospital, I was directed back to pre-op to visit John prior to surgery. Before I saw him, I was briefed on the injuries sustained as well as the initial prognosis. John had fractured his thoracic spine and had nearly lost his left leg. Both injuries were so devastating that the neurosurgeons and orthopedic surgeons had to consult several times to decide what to repair first, the spine or the leg. If the spine were chosen, there was an increased probability of losing the leg, and if the leg, an increased probability of permanent paralysis. As I spoke with John, he was fully aware of the grave situation. He said to me, "I fractured my spine and I think I may be paralyzed, but I'll be all right."

Several months of rehabilitation left John with the ability to return to his regular activities, including his career and working out. Only this time he was paralyzed from the waist down. But John never missed a beat. Not once did I hear him ask, "Why me?" Nor did he send out announcements for a pity party. He simply would say, "This is the deck of cards I've been dealt, and I'll play my hand the best that I can."

Today John is in excellent shape and looks a good 7-10 years younger than most his age. Maybe it's just me, but when someone like John can find the time to take care of himself, it makes me feel guilty for complaining about going to the gym. If you think you're short on time, try making your every move from a wheel chair.

Celebrate your gift of a fully functioning body. And care for that gift wisely! Start by developing good habits and crowding out the bad ones.

* * *

"After three months, I have a new outlook on life and feel empowered to make changes. I also see the results I have been looking for. I am ready to start the next chapter in my life feeling healthy, strong, and alive.

"I recommend this program to anyone wanting to improve his or her health physical and mental. You will emerge transformed and be able to reclaim the healthy body you deserve."

Nancy Heinke
San Antonio, TX

"I had reached an age where managing my weight, hormones and general health and wellbeing was becoming an increasing struggle—one which I was not winning.

"Aside from losing weight and improving my body and health in general, my sleep is deep, restorative and refreshing, my blood pressure has gone down to a healthy level, my energy levels are much higher than before, I seem to be thinking more clearly, I feel confident, my outlook is happy, enthusiastic, positive and optimistic, I just feel good. Really, really good.

"It is wonderful! I would recommend this program to anyone who is serious about improving his or her physical and mental wellbeing and health."

Vicki Schwartz
Beorne, TX

"I started the Reclaim 24 wellness program 1 day after my 49th birthday. My overall health complaints included: Can't lose weight; no energy; extreme fatigue; neck pain and numbness in the arms and hands I was taking an average of 6 Advil per day, with high blood pressure averaging 140/95 mm Hg while taking 3 BP medications.

"My official results as of 4/22/09 in a nutshell: I have lost 38 lbs; my energy is restored; I sleep through the night soundly; I have significantly reduced pain to the point that I no longer take Advil or other pain relievers, and I am completely off BP meds.

"I just listened, followed their recipe, and now I have the proof that it works!"

Hugs with Love,
Darla Rucka
San Antonio, TX

6: You *Can* Succeed with Weight Loss And Fitness!

In the back of your mind you may have a lingering fear of failure about this program. Like most, at some time you've undoubtedly attempted to accomplish some change regarding your health and appearance. You may have even achieved a short-lived level of accomplishment and satisfaction. Did you fail because you lacked discipline or purpose? Was the exercise program too extensive and time consuming? Or was the diet too restrictive and impossible to maintain?

Chances are all of these factors played a role in your failure(s). If you've followed any of the typical fitness and diet programs we see being taught today, it doesn't surprise me that you failed to reach your goals. From infomercials promising results from the use of their newest "Ab Buster" to health stores selling "quick fix" pills, Americans are literally bombarded with so much garbage that they just give up. Do any of these gadgets or pills actually work? Do you really know anyone who has transformed his or her body using this stuff?

Of course you don't. That's because this junk is manufactured and marketed for the sole purpose of making a quick profit. Not that making a profit is wrong, but selling a product that doesn't stand up to its claims is. Yet these master marketers continue to fool the public year after year, producing new and better "Ab Busters" and more potent pills guaranteed to make you look like those young, tight-bodied models featured on the commercials and on the packaging materials.

Did you ever take time to evaluate the likelihood that these models look like they do strictly by using that silly stuff? I have some heart-breaking news for you: not only do they work out regularly using weight resistance exercises, they also eat extremely healthy diets. Fitness is their living and provides them with their income. What they don't do is waste precious time using any of the worthless items they promote. Master marketers know that Americans are gullible impulse buyers and are always looking for quick fixes for problems developed over a long time.

Enough. This time around, let's move forward to discuss ways to succeed with weight loss and fitness. Oh, but before we continue, why not put this book down. Look under your bed, in the closet, or perhaps in the attic or garage, to locate any pieces of "fitness" junk you once

45

purchased at a time when you were naïve. Now take that stuff to the curb for trash pickup. Let this symbolic and practical gesture serve to "make room" in your imagination and your life for an approach that works and brings success!

Finding a Qualified Mentor: the First Crucial Step

Think back to a time when you succeeded at some much-desired goal, whether a major test taken in high school or college, or maybe some athletic event. In your present career, perhaps you surpassed your best sales month or successfully conquered a seemingly mountainous trial or problem. In the majority of cases where success appears, you also find a mentor or coach.

Successful athletes frequently credit their coaches before praising their own abilities. Top salespeople are always able to quickly name one or more mentors responsible for their success. The quickest, surest way to find success is to first find a creditable mentor. These are the people who have experienced the trials and difficulties of achievement within the field of your interest. They have already learned the hard lessons that *precede* success and probably have the gray hair (or no hair) to prove it.

You've probably heard the famous Thomas Edison quote, "I have not failed. I've just found 10,000 ways that won't work." By persistence, trial, and discard, a qualified mentor or coach will have found out how to achieve the goal you seek in ways that will save you time, effort, and unnecessary hardships. This is the coach you want in your corner!

I know it's not easy for "rugged individualists" to accept mentorship. They are the ones who typically say, "Leave me alone, I want to figure it all out for myself." This country was created mostly on the efforts of rugged individualists, so that kind of thinking has its place.

Nonetheless, this is the point where I ask you, Mr. or Ms. Rugged Individual, to *suspend your natural leaning for the duration of my 12-week "proof of concept."* I'm asking you to take a few risks in relying on my method of coaching. Just let go for a while so you can clear away the cobwebs of old.

If we're smart, we embrace the Edisons of the world when it makes sense. In this way, we avoid many of the pitfalls we surely would experience retracing the same path on our own. Even more importantly, mentors show us some of the trials that we might face down the road. Knowing ahead of time what to expect allows us to prepare and pass through such trials with greater confidence (and often the mentor's inspiration). Of course, we'll make fresh mistakes on our own, but the least we can do is avoid traveling well-worn paths strewn with the bodies of go-it-aloners. So, unless you're one of those people who simply *must* go it alone and take *all* the hard knocks, learn from someone else when you can. You'll find more time for new adventures in your life!

Here's the thing. If the goal of health and fitness warrants a high priority in your life, there will be trials and difficulties. You can take that knowledge to the bank. You know this if you've ever achieved anything of importance. It's through such trials that we develop our character, confidence, true humility, and self-respect.

A Qualified Mentor Will Know How to Unleash the Goal-Achieving Powers of the Mind

Napoleon Hill (*Think & Grow Rich*), Tony Robbins (*Unlimited Power*), Maxwell Maltz, M.D., (*Psycho-Cybernetics*), and Jack Nicklaus (*Jack Nicklaus: My Story*) are all known as successful mentors who harvested the *power of thought* to make dramatic changes both in their lives and the lives of others. **They learned how potent it is to displace one's fear of failure with a tenacious and vivid end-goal picture; to doggedly embrace in one's mind—and emotions—the <u>desired</u> end result rather than the undesired one!** And they, like so many in human history, have freely shared their discoveries about this amazing power. But so few takers step forward to embrace the powers they have within themselves. What's going on here?

Why Do So Many People Dwell in the Failure Habit?

People refuse the gifts of growth and achievement for many reasons. Going into all of them isn't my purpose. I'll just summarize by saying the *primary* reason people fail is that they expect to fail! Failure is their familiar companion. They often think of past failures and habitually picture those failures in their minds and "relive them" within the solar plexus. They believe others are also doomed to failure unless they get lucky. At

> "Human beings always act and feel and perform in accordance with what they imagine to be true about themselves and their environment." – Maxwell Maltz, *Psycho-Cybernetics*

47

the bottom of it all, these people are comfortable with failure, much like being comfortable with a well-worn pair of sneakers.

With this negative picturing going on day in and day out, they unwittingly announce to the world that they hold failure dear, even though they immediately deny it when challenged. And they predictably reward themselves with failure over and over again! As each new reward comes rolling in, they are further vindicated in their belief that failure is their lot. Could life speak to them any more clearly than that?

How powerful, this negative self-prophecy!

The Peculiar Power of Pernicious Predictors

There's a lot more than just negative self-prophecy going on with this failure challenge. Let me introduce you to Pernicious Patty. She, and so many like her (men and women alike), is here to help you fail even beyond any failure you might thrust on yourself.

People absolutely love to predict—even though they're hardly ever right about anything important (but even a stopped clock is right twice a day). The dark side of all this is that, with precious few exceptions—you and me for sure—Pernicious Patty spews predictions for two reasons: first, to feel self-important, and second, to lord power over others. Strangely, there always seems to be an audience willing to listen to her. And this audience is often foolish enough to "buy in" to her predictive imagery with little, if any, conscious resistance or consideration. It's quite peculiar how people seem to leave the doors to their minds wide open to Patty's garbage. They must think it's harmless. But it's not.

One minute Pernicious Patty is claiming the ability to make divine utterances. The next she is telling us how the stock market must inevitably move. A minute after that she is telling us that somebody's marriage won't last. How long do you think it will be before she is predicting you won't be able to meet your weight loss and fitness goals?

Patty, always ready and eager to inject prediction venom into a victim's consciousness, expects others to fail and is adept at creating the negative imagery to help them do so.

If Susceptible Sam has yet to learn self-protection from a Pernicious Patty injection, the next thing you know *his subconscious mind is adopting Patty's failure imagery, lock, stock, and barrel.* Shortly, we'll find Patty as happy as a sow in a mud puddle because she sees that Sam is failing, just as she predicted. What talent!

Of course, Patty wants to make sure her talent doesn't go unnoticed, so the words, "I told you so," readily pass through her lips to remind Sam of her pernicious predictive power. Little does Patty understand that she is personally responsible for damaging Susceptible Sam's mind through reckless, intrusive "programming"—but that's another story. What we need to understand is that we're not going to be able to eject every Pernicious Patty from the planet any time soon. It's truly Sam's duty to build immunity from her failure injections.

How the Subconscious Mind Works to Help or Hurt You

One can write volumes about the subconscious mind. I only want to cover a few important points about it in a non-technical way. These points are *all* relevant to your success with the *Reclaim 24* Action Plan, as well as other goals in your life. At the heart of it all, you must understand how the subconscious mind works tirelessly behind the scenes to help you bring into your life *what you've come to expect through the persistent pictures you hold in your mind's eye.* This includes pictures of accomplishment, failure, and everything in between. These pictures, of course, do not have to be strictly visual. "Feeling" pictures are just as potent.

If upon reading the next few pages you find that you already understand what I'm covering here, congratulations! You're one in ten thousand. Do share what you know with others as appropriate, just as our "mentors" have shared with us.

Our Robotic Companion, the Subconscious Mind

The subconscious mind—often called the "subconscious" for short—is powerfully efficient yet blindly reactive in its stealthy, computer-like responses. Working in the background 24/7, it "watches and listens" for opportunities to support the conscious mind in carrying out anything routine. As part of this support, when it perceives that the conscious mind is engaging in some form of patterned decision-making, it records the pattern in its hidden memory. Repetition of a pattern signals the subconscious to convert or "harden" the results of conscious decision-making into automatic behavior or responses. The more the repetition, the more "grooved" the automatic behavior becomes. Recording grooves become especially deep when the emotional charges of pleasure or pain accompany your decision imagery.

So, the conscious mind makes decisions (or often "thinks" it does) while the subconscious "learns" about chosen or expected outcomes so it can supportively repeat those outcomes. Without this companionship between the conscious and subconscious parts of the mind, we could never learn to walk, ride a bicycle, drive to work, play a musical instrument, or dish out clever repartees to intrusive mothers-in-law.

Yet, unlike the conscious mind, the subconscious has no ability to discriminate or make value judgments. In fact, it can't decide anything. It just learns and repeats what the conscious mind has "taught" it to repeat. What you need most to remember about this lack of discrimination is that the subconscious has no power to *evaluate* whether or not its repetitive actions are holistically good for you. It supports you in failure as well as accomplishment if that's what you "teach" it to do with your repetitive decisions and pictured expectations. Bottom line: We choose between failure and accomplishment with our dominant, internal imagery and behavior patterns.

Now, recall that—as a built-in biological tendency—the human organism is programmed to blindly move toward physical and emotional pleasure and away from pain. If you don't assess what you're doing for its long-term value in your life, you'll probably allow holistically poor behaviors to become deeply imbedded in your subconscious to the point where you'll stop discriminating at all. For example, if you teach your subconscious that you have a definite preference for being a couch potato, then taking care of your health recedes further and further into the background until it all but disappears. Then, only the physical and emotional pain of poor health gets you thinking consciously again! But sometimes it's too late.

Feelin' Groovy?

Seldom do people understand how powerful the grooves in the subconscious mind can become. But here's a common example that demonstrates this grooving power—an example that I'll bet you've experienced in similar ways many times.

Let's suppose that your boss said something obnoxious that disturbed you yesterday. Now you're playing it back in your mind. The more you play it, the less you like it. Suddenly you think of a clever rebuke you could have used in the heat of the moment but didn't think of at the time.

So now you're picturing yourself dishing out this clever rebuke instead of taking your boss's verbal assault on the chin, as you did. This imaginary rebuke is your secret way of emotionally "getting even" with your boss without your getting into trouble. You've become a "Walter Mitty" kind of hero because your verbal cleverness has won the day—at least in your imagination. And so you replay this rebuke for a few days because you get heroic pleasure with each repetition. And it almost surely has quite an emotional charge that goes along with it. With time, however, the whole incident and your gut reaction to it begin to fade.

Then one day not too far in the future, your flesh-and-blood boss walks into your office and those magic trigger words that riled you once before come sliding off his tongue again. This time, just like one of Pavlov's dogs salivating at the ringing of a bell, you immediately release that practiced, clever rebuke. But wait! That rebuke was intended only for the secret chambers of your imagination, not the real world! But alas, you watch in horror as it leaps from your lips, just as you had practiced it in your imagination.

You have, in fact, been trapped by your deeply grooved subconscious mind! You just can't stop it once triggered. You stand by and watch helplessly as the words gush forth and your next annual raise falls off the table. Then, after the smoke clears and you're alone once again, you shake your head and wonder why in the world you can't control your tongue. But you'd be wrong wondering about that. In truth, you controlled yourself just as you had imagined! After all, what's a good, non-discriminating subconscious mind for?

And THAT, dear reader, is one powerful example of the subconscious mind in action. It's not just an abstract entity that intellectuals talk about. No, it's right here in your face. And constantly. So, we all need to come to grips with its "groovy" behavior and learn how best to take advantage of it rather than have it bite us in the rear (and maybe the paycheck).

Warning: The Subconscious Mind Can't Comprehend Negation!

Another fascinating thing you learn about the subconscious mind and its native ignorance is that it ignores negation—"don'ts" and "nots." It can only accept the picture or imagery you're flashing before it—*not its absence or undesirability*. Don'ts and nots dwell only in the logical part of the mind and not in the imaginative part that makes pictures. In truth, don'ts and nots are kicked to the curb on the way to the command center! They don't register upon the subconscious.

As a familiar example of this subconscious "shortcoming" in action, do not imagine a pink elephant gleefully dancing on its hind legs while wearing a flower-embroidered apron. My "do not" command didn't help you cancel out the picture, did it? You simply had to picture the pink elephant in your imagination before you could comprehend what you shouldn't be picturing in your imagination. By then, however, it was too late! Your subconscious took note of the dancing, apron-wearing pink elephant and stored it in memory. Do that often enough and the video clip will play ever more easily and clearly.

But there is something sneaky that can be going on behind the scenes with don'ts and nots. I mentioned earlier that emotions of pleasure or pain tend to groove images into the subconscious more strongly. The fact is that conscious or unconscious fears usually accompany images of experiences we are trying to avoid in our lives. This just grooves the unwanted imagery more deeply, despite our internal don'ts and nots.

The lesson, of course, is that telling yourself over and over again *not* to engage in some undesirable habit just grooves a picture of the undesired habit into your subconscious mind. The "not" gets lost. Therefore, the subconscious, in doing its job, tries to make the habit you're attempting to avoid evermore easy to repeat! This is one of the reasons preachers of moral behavior so often fail miserably at what they preach to others *not* to do. Then, the next thing you know, you find them publicly grieving for having failed in their own behavior and gotten caught. If they understood how the subconscious mind works, they would preach about what everyone *should* be doing! Now that would be a refreshing change.

Bottom line: **Create imagery of things that you *want* to happen. That's the only way to combat negative imagery—by displacing it. And that's one of the secrets of the ages that qualified mentors teach.**

Programming the Subconscious from Within

Just as the subconscious doesn't recognize or process negation, neither does it recognize distinctions between images received via the outer senses and those presented to it by your imagination. The subconscious treats it all the same. In fact, today, many athletes—*once they already know the correct physical movements or actions—*

"practice" their specialties in their mind's eye and get almost identical results to physical practice. Research has proven conclusively that this imaginative approach works.

Of course, first-class athletes aren't the only ones who can benefit from this subconscious skill. You can, too.

So take regular daydream time to "practice" your goals (and steps to achieving them) by picturing them already achieved in your imagination and your enjoying them. This imaginative "reinforcement" works because the subconscious doesn't give a hoot from whence it gets its stimuli for action. It supports you just the same. But it also works because of the seldom-discussed principle of connected minds.

Adopting the Principle of Connected Minds For Creative "Team Building"

Subconscious minds seem to be connected in ways we can't see or measure with physical instruments. Maybe they are connected by the laws of quantum mechanics; or maybe by the nature of Jung's universal unconscious. But exactly *how* subconscious minds connect with each other isn't so important at all. What *is* important for you to know is this: SUBCONSCIOUS MINDS INFLUENCE EACH OTHER, OFTEN AT GREAT DISTANCES.

This influence-at-a-distance allows your most private, creative expectations to reach out across the world and rally dozens, hundreds, maybe thousands of other subconscious minds to cooperate with your "programmed" intentions when your intentions are compatible with theirs. Even life's "laws of chance" begin to line up for you when you decide to accept the gifts offered to you by the inherent powers of the mind and the hidden universal laws that influence those powers. All of a sudden synchronicity[2] and serendipity[3] start breaking out all over the place for your benefit! It's a wonder to behold.

Experience tells me that most people don't have a clue about the principle of connected minds even though much psychological research

---

[2] Coincidence of events that seem to be meaningfully related, conceived in the theory of Carl Jung as an explanatory principle on the same order as causality. (*The American Heritage Dictionary of the English Language,* Third Edition Copyright © 1992 by Houghton Mifflin Company.)
[3] The faculty of making fortunate discoveries by accident. (Ibid)

and human experience strongly support it. The fact is that most people use the enormous creative power of their subconscious minds to build fences around themselves—like chickens restricted to pecking away in a fenced-in barnyard. Yet, they have the power of an eagle to soar freely on heavenly wind currents where they can spot opportunities at great distances. But they don't soar. Instead, they place pictures of limitation in their minds—barnyard fences. And sure enough, those minds deliver on the pictures! So the chicken-pecking continues.

Of course, this principle of connected minds has its skeptics. If you're wise, you won't allow skeptics to inject you with their pernicious doubt, for once they do, the action of your subconscious mind in embracing doubt helps to make it your reality, too! See how it works?

The practical working principles of human creativity reveal themselves more easily to those who don't insist on "scientific proclamation" to legitimize the principles. Don't shut yourself off from the gifts of the Universe because others do so with pride and conviction. Instead, pay attention to people like the mentors I cited earlier. They won't lead you astray. Do welcome, wholeheartedly, such supportive minds so that you can fully benefit from the *Reclaim 24* lifestyle program I'm offering here. Once you learn how to do it, you are able to apply the principles *in every area of your life*. So think of *Reclaim 24* as a step into your world of unbounded creative achievement.

A Nutshell Summary of the Subconscious Mind's Influence

Your subconscious mind blindly accepts your dominant thoughts and imagery. It knows nothing of good, bad, right, or wrong. It simply accepts information, in the same way a computer does. And when a pattern is established, it plays that information back in the form of physical, emotional, or mental behavior. The more deeply the pattern is set through reinforcement and emotional charge, the more automatic the resulting behavior.

> "Dream lofty dreams, and as you dream, so shall you become. The greatest achievement was at first and for a time a dream." – James Allen, *As a Man Thinketh*

If you truly believe your destiny is to be poverty-stricken, your subconscious mind will guide your actions to achieve exactly what you've pictured—to go broke and stay that way. Not only that, it summons the resources of other subconscious minds around the Universe to help you stay broke. You'll even find yourself physically running into some of the people who own those subconscious minds, day after day!

If you're leery of the truth behind this principle, just look at your friends and acquaintances who are doing well in comparison to those who are not. Generally, those who seem to easily excel have a good attitude and a confident spirit. They know where they are going and believe they can continue to prosper and reach new goals. They believe in outcomes that bring pleasure and happiness. In contrast, those who seemingly never change and continue to struggle also believe in outcomes; they just believe in negative outcomes and pallid goals.

So the principle is clear: if you fail to monitor your thoughts and images, other people's thoughts and images will intrusively find their way into your subconscious mind. Because most human beings are largely negative in their outlook, the images they project to you are most often wholeheartedly negative. So select your thoughts, imagery, and mentors carefully, and you'll be well on the way to altering your future for the better.

Jumpstart Your Subconscious with Positive Visualization

Napoleon Hill stated in his book "Think & Grow Rich" that the task of controlling one's thoughts takes great effort. It's not easy to control your mind when it's constantly babbling on, especially when you're trying to fall asleep at the end of a busy day. With the mind constantly talking, you can be left with little quiet time. To shut this jibber jabber out takes a conscious and concerted effort.

If you don't make the effort to deliberately condition (or recondition) your subconscious mind with constructive imagery, then random, meaningless thoughts and imagery fill the void.

By now you know that the subconscious can be a welcome sidekick if it's given good patterns to soak up and automatically play back at the right time. On the other hand, if it's handed garbage, such as "I'm getting old," or "I'm a failure at weight control," or "My mother-in-law wears army boots," it just spews back the garbage handed to it and impacts our behaviors accordingly. This is the reason so many people stumble through life without any real direction. Year after year they allow their subconscious minds to soak up meaningless conversation, negative thoughts and projections, and persistent, profitless behaviors that add little if any value to their lives.

On the other hand, if you constantly see in your mind's eye an end result that you desire, you accept it as real, and you tie your feelings to it, all the other characteristics for success such as discipline, action, and perseverance start becoming automatic.

By frequently visualizing your desired end-result in a relaxed way (better health, toned body), it programs your subconscious mind into accepting your visualized pattern. The unusual powers of the subconscious mind then begin to *automatically* organize themselves around your continually reinforced image and any associated physical practices. This changes your behavior and a new habit is born. Your conscious mind even conforms its decision making to subconsciously influenced behaviors. After a while, your decisions—if you need to make them at all—begin to feel effortless because the subconscious has taken over.

It's no different from learning to ride a bicycle. You start out by seeing yourself riding, and your subconscious adopts the picture. Then you "practice," which gives your subconscious the opportunity to align nervous system "trials" and your musculoskeletal system with the embedded picture. Soon the picture and your nervous system behavior "become one" and you're a bicyclist! Maybe you never thought of it this way, but being able to ride a bicycle is a habit that starts with imagery.

Please remember this: The imagery we place in our minds is a choice. The dominant feelings that we walk around with are a choice. I choose to talk about the things that I think you want instead of those you don't want. Please be a taker! Please be one of those unusual few who accepts the gifts of growth offered by others.

PART II:
YOUR RECLAIM 24, 12-WEEK ACTION PLAN

Learn how to exercise smarter, not harder. My approach is an exact science that gets you burning fat 24/7. I take you through baby steps that will prevent you from making the mistake of over-exercising. You'll no longer have to spend 30 to 60 minutes on a treadmill, which can actually work against you. With *Reclaim 24*, you become a master at transforming your body and spend no more than 35–40 minutes at exercise three times per week.

What's more, you don't need a PhD in nutrition to understand how to choose foods that not only energize and nourish but also activate fat-burning hormones instead of fat-storing hormones. You simply must experience the *Reclaim 24* food-choice and meal-scheduling process to understand why my system works and others don't. It's all about simplicity and a strong, scientific foundation. You can even buy most of your foods from a conventional supermarket if you shop carefully.

7: Resistance Training *Demythified!*

Resistance training is one of my areas of expertise. Not only have I done the research necessary to help you avoid being misled by the myths that pervade this area of fitness, I also live it. I know the current and leading-edge science about resistance training, as well as all the official "long words" that prevail in this discipline. But I'm going to avoid getting too academic or technical since that will *not* help you get into the shape you want. Most of what you need to know is simple. So let's jump in!

The Importance of Weight Training for Optimal Health

Unfortunately, many ignore resistance or weight training when devising their exercise plan, thinking they don't want to "bulk up." But gaining more muscle through resistance exercises is an integral part of any well-rounded fitness program, especially if you want to lose weight—and doubly so as the calendar years add up.

You should know, however, that weight training for wellness is not about vanity. The intensity of your resistance training can achieve a number of beneficial changes in the molecular, enzymatic, hormonal, and chemical systems in your body.

Train Smarter, Not Harder!

When it comes to resistance training (including weight training), more isn't better. Time and again I witness individuals spending hours in the gym, five to six days a week, performing marathon numbers of sets[4] in the futile attempt to gain muscle and body tone. I say futile because, month after month and year after year, these people rarely change. Yet they continue to believe that if a little is good, then more must be better. If they would only reflect on the time and effort they've spent over the years, they would conclude that their training methods must be flawed. But few people seek competent advice for using resistance training to

---

[4] In bodybuilding jargon, a "set" is a repetitive movement, without rest, using the same equipment. Each set targets a specific body part or muscle group, such as the legs. So, in essence, the word "set" is short for the phrase, "set of repetitions." Effective workouts may require more than one set of repetitions for each targeted body part.

grow muscle mass or develop better body tone. Nor do they personally research the methods they use, or even try random changes to see if they can stumble across a better workout.

If you've been seeking advice on exercise routines, I commend you. However, if you're getting your advice from popular muscle magazines—both the male and female versions—you've probably already discovered that most of them follow the "more is better concept." You have read that so-and-so pro bodybuilder or fitness queen performs four different exercises at five sets apiece per body part (for example, the chest). You think, "Well gosh, if it works for him or her, it will surely work for me!" Sorry.

With the possible exception of athletes using performance-enhancing drugs, the more-is-better approach leads to overtraining—the number one reason body shapers and bodybuilders fail to progress. Performance-enhancing drugs often get results for very heavy trainers because they allow athletes to recuperate more quickly and efficiently following a stressful workout. These athletes, therefore, don't suffer from the tear-down effects of overtraining (but they may suffer from the side effects of performance drugs).

Every once in a while, an athlete blessed with superior genes comes along and is able to get spectacular results from heavy workouts year after year without using drugs. But it hardly ever happens. And you're not likely to be one with such superior genes or you'd know it. The general rule is that long-term physique builders *who follow persistently heavy workout schedules* must resort to stress-adapting drugs if they want superior results. Not a pretty picture.

But knowing what research has shown about the deleterious effects of overtraining, I must even question the results achieved by genetically gifted athletes. I wonder what kind of results they would have gotten if they had allowed for more recuperation and had trained smarter? Would they have been able to achieve even better results if they had spent less time in the gym and more time resting? I think so.

Actually, I'm confident that they would have at least achieved the same physique while cutting in half the time spent in the gym. And as I mentioned earlier, this extra time could certainly be better spent adopting more of the personal lifestyle behaviors identified in the four crucial categories of wellness (page 25). What good is a dynamite exterior without an interesting, mature, capable, loving interior to go along with it?

Differences in Muscle Development Between the Sexes

You need to understand the proven principles of muscle development whether your goal is to achieve a well-muscled physique or simply to lose a few pounds to get that toned appearance so many desire. The physiologic concepts remain the same. It's muscle growth (both size and density) that ultimately shapes our bodies, speeds our metabolism, and enables us to readily maintain our desired contours and dimensions.

Now if you're a woman you might easily be thinking, "I don't want to put on muscle and get bulky like some of those fitness girls." Please understand that simply won't happen. Women who build muscle easily are the rare exception and not the rule.

First, your hormone make-up won't allow it. Although you do produce the muscle-building hormone, testosterone, your level is minute—only a fraction of that produced by men. Plus, your muscles are naturally smaller than men's muscles to start with. Without high levels of testosterone, your development is quite limited, at least in terms of "bulking up." Those bulky women body builders shown in some fitness magazines have usually had help from supplements or steroids. Moreover, they have been training—in bodybuilding rather than fitness—for years if not decades.

You are, however, more than capable of stimulating muscle growth and thus building a shapely, well-toned body much as so many female celebrities are doing these days. Now, what woman would truly be concerned about developing a little bit too much firmness in her backside?

So, for the last time, let's discard that "bulking" excuse and realize that resistance training is mandatory if a wonderfully contoured body is part of your fitness goal. And one more thing. Remember that, as you add muscle, you become stronger and firmer, you increase bone density (which may help prevent osteoporosis later in life), and your metabolism increases, enhancing your ability to burn off unwanted fat.

If you're a man, you must also understand that "bulking up" isn't so easy, either. If you've been weight training for several years, you know what I'm talking about. Although you have moderate to high levels of naturally produced testosterone circulating throughout your body, you may lack some of the genetics required to build a world-class physique. In fact, most men don't have this potential and for this reason should pay strict attention to this next point:

> ### *If you want to maximize your individual potential, you must avoid overtraining—at all costs.*

As I mentioned earlier, overtraining is the number one reason so many people fail to progress.

The Need for High-Intensity, Short-Duration Workouts

The resistance training aspect of the *Reclaim 24* Action Plan is based on the principle of stimulating muscle groups with high levels of intensity to make those groups adapt to the higher stress. This means you must consistently attempt to induce a higher level of stress than the previous workout. This forces muscles to change their structure, to grow. If the level of intensity remains the same, muscles eventually adapt and no longer respond with growth. The good thing about performing an exercise at a high-intensity level is that it takes fewer *sets*[5] to stimulate muscles for maximum growth. That means workouts are short and sweet.

The principle here is simple. Your muscles respond and grow under high-intensity stress much better than low-intensity stress. But if you overdo high intensity by working out too long or performing too many sets, new muscle development stops and injuries take over. In fact:

> ### *It's even possible for your muscles to shrink because too much stress creates a hormonal condition that converts muscle into fuel to protect the body from the additional stress. And there goes all your efforts to build muscle!*

On the other hand, if workout intensity is too low, your muscles may never get the full stimulus they need and won't fully develop, even with plenty of time in the gym.

---

[5] Remember, a "set" means a number of repetitive movements without rest, using the same equipment.

You can easily see how this principle works with professional athletes. Compare the sport of sprinting with that of long-distance running, for example. Sprinters have lean, well-muscled physiques (both men and women). Their workouts consist of high-intensity, short-duration routines. In contrast, when you look at long distance or marathon runners—those who typically run over 100 miles per week at slow speeds (relative to sprinters)—you see they have somewhat soft, stringy muscles with little definition. They look absolutely nothing like the athletes who run 100-yard dashes. In truth, marathon runners are *severely overtrained,* which has been verified by objective tests. Further, their blood levels of antioxidants rank just below smokers, which isn't at all a good sign!

The Facts about Overtraining

If you wish to develop the body you dream of, you must avoid overtraining at all costs. To make this crystal clear, I'll stress that overtraining is the act of working a muscle or group of muscles beyond what is needed to induce a maximum stimulus for growth. That means you should focus only on performing a *quality* set or sets of exercises rather than increasing the number of sets.

Earlier I talked about the deleterious effects of overtraining or over-exercise. For the doubters and non-believers, I'll now go into detail as to why overtraining is a problem. It's all about stress and the hormone cortisol.

Cortisol is an important hormone in the body. It is secreted by the adrenal glands and involved in the following functions and more:

- Proper glucose metabolism
- Regulation of blood pressure
- Insulin release for blood sugar maintenance
- Immune function
- Inflammatory response

A high level of physical or mental stress causes fat, protein, and carbohydrates, along with epinephrine and a number of other endocrine hormones, to be rapidly mobilized in order for you to take quick action against the stressor (the well-known "fight or flight" response to stress). During this mobilization, cortisol and adrenaline increase while DHEA (Dehydro-epiandrosterone) and testosterone decrease.

Normally, cortisol is present in the body at higher levels in the morning and at its lowest level at night. The fight-or-flight response to stress isn't the only reason cortisol is secreted into the bloodstream. It is also responsible for several other stress-related changes in the body.

Small increases of cortisol have some positive effects in the body:

- A quick burst of energy for survival purposes
- Heightened memory function
- A burst of increased immunity
- Lower sensitivity to pain
- The maintenance of homeostasis[6] in the body

While cortisol is an important and helpful part of the body's response to stress, it's also important for the body to activate its *relaxation response* following a stressful event. This allows the body's functions to return to normal.

Unfortunately, in our current high-stress culture, the body's stress response ramps up so often that it doesn't have a chance to return to normal. This results in a state of chronic stress with higher and more prolonged levels of cortisol being present in the bloodstream. Moreover, you should know that high-intensity exercise and prolonged exercise both increase cortisol levels. This means that overtraining creates chronic stress in the body along with high, prolonged levels of cortisol!

Cortisol levels remain elevated for about 2 hours following an exercise session, since exercise is a stressor. Therefore, prolonged exercise sessions, or repeated sessions without appropriate rest between the sessions, results in chronic, elevated cortisol. Additionally, poor diet, inadequate supplementation, and lack of rest in general also play key roles in cortisol secretion.

A *chronically* elevated cortisol level causes your body to enter a state of constant muscle breakdown and suppressed immune function, increasing your risk of illness and injury while cannibalizing muscle tissue. That's right. **Chronically high cortisol levels shrink muscle tissue.** Cortisol has a catabolic (muscle breakdown) effect on tissue and is associated with a decrease in anabolic (muscle growth) hormones like IGF-1 and GH. Because of this, we've learned that minimizing cortisol

---

[6] The body's natural tendency to maintain—or attempt to maintain—an internal stability or balance. The organ systems of the body do this by coordinating biological responses that automatically compensate for environmental changes.

levels is ideal for an athlete if he or she wishes to achieve tissue growth and positive adaptations to exercise training.

Another negative outcome of too much cortisol is increased abdominal fat. Aside from appearance frustrations, increased abdominal fat is associated with a greater number of health problems than fat deposited in other areas of the body. This happens because abdominal fat can secrete dangerous hormones. Some of the health problems associated with excess stomach fat are heart attacks, strokes, and a poor cholesterol profile that can lead to other health problems.

Still other negative effects of too much cortisol are:

- Reduction in athletic performance because of fatigue and inflammation
- Reduction in ligament health
- Poorer sleep quality
- Mood swings
- Reduced sex drive
- Decreased bone density
- Slowed wound healing
- Impaired cognitive performance
- Suppressed thyroid function
- Imbalanced in blood sugar such as hyperglycemia
- Higher blood pressure
- Lowered immunity and other inflammatory responses in the body

Cortisol secretion varies among individuals. People are biologically "wired" to react differently to stress. One person may secrete higher levels of cortisol than another in the same situation. Studies have also shown that people who secrete higher levels of cortisol in response to stress also tend to eat more than people who secrete less cortisol. They also eat food higher in carbohydrates. If you're more sensitive to stress, it's especially important for you to learn stress-management techniques as well as adopting a low-stress lifestyle to the degree possible.

How Do I Know if My Cortisol Levels Are High?

Mood swings, lack of motivation to train, loss of muscle, and loss of appetite are all symptoms of an elevated cortisol level. Sound familiar? That's right: It's the overtraining syndrome!

If you are not taking steps to modulate your cortisol, you are breaking down your muscle, storing fat, and getting sick, none of which make sense for someone interested in wellness!

A more scientific approach is to have your testosterone/cortisol or IGF-1/cortisol levels tested. A suppressed ratio of either IGF or testosterone over cortisol is a sure sign of decreased exercise capacity and overtraining. There is also strong evidence that an athlete who exercises in a carbohydrate-depleted state experiences greater increases in cortisol. Decreased frequency of menstrual periods in women (amenorrhea) has been linked to insufficient energy availability. That, in turn, triggers a stress-hormone response and suppresses estrogen and progesterone.

How Does Cortisol Affect My Endurance?

It is only with chronically elevated cortisol levels that your performance suffers, but the effect is dramatic. Because excess cortisol suppresses your immune system, you have a greater risk of upper respiratory infections. Of course, as mentioned, your body enters a catabolic state—breaking down muscle and storing fat.

In addition to reducing your muscle and getting sick, suppressed testosterone means suppressed recovery. Aerobic and anaerobic muscle fibers need time to repair and recover from hard workouts to improve their capacity to exercise. Elevated cortisol and suppressed testosterone do not allow you to maximize your recovery, leading to slower performance gains. Additionally, amenorrhea in women and low testosterone in men may increase risk for stress fractures.

How Can I Modulate Cortisol?

You can modulate your cortisol production through rest, nutrition, and supplementation. First, since repeated bouts of exercise cause chronic, elevated cortisol, it is crucial to get plenty of rest between workouts. You get your best results, by far, with a day or two of rest between workouts.

Bottom line: Once you've completed the number of sets to be outlined in the *Reclaim 24* Workout of the next chapter, **you need to discontinue exercising that particular muscle group for the remainder of the session.** *If you press ahead with additional sets, it means either you did not fatigue yourself with the required number of* *sets, or you're simply choosing to ignore this rule—at your peril.* Then cortisol becomes your enemy instead of your friend.

The Physiology of Muscle Development

To further help you avoid the temptation to perform extra sets, I'll explain the physiology of muscle development.

For a muscle to change, it must first be subject to a stimulus such as weight-resistance exercise. This stress or stimulus results in micro-trauma to the individual fibers (myofibrils) that make up that muscle. When the body repairs these micro-tears—a typical process for muscles—it leads to a stronger and more developed muscle. If the repair process is hindered in any way, the full potential for growth is minimized and the results are disappointing.

When does the repair process take place? Well it sure doesn't take place while you are forcing additional sets upon a muscle group that you've already stressed to the hilt!

> *Muscle growth and repair occur only when you are resting. No rest equals no growth!*

This following point is strange but true. When a muscle has been fully stressed but not overstressed, *rest is the closest thing you can get to using anabolic steroids for muscle growth.* The effects are quite similar. So, if you want those muscles to respond to the hard work you put in at the gym or at home, you simply *must* allow plenty of time for rest, which even includes taking an occasional nap.

Naps are anabolic (tissue building) in nature and work wonders for mental recuperation as well. Rest also means staying away from the gym between workouts. You use these rest days to take care of other life matters or to simply enjoy some leisure time.

Please remember the reason you're reading this book. You're unhappy with past results and are hoping this program will be your answer. It *will* be your answer if you trust me and allow me to serve as your mentor. Follow the program! Although there are countless things in life that I don't know much about, this topic isn't one of them. This is an area of expertise for me. Please take advantage of that.

The Importance of Resistance Training as You Age

I'm sure it's no surprise to you that as we age our muscles want to shrink, which decreases strength and increases the likelihood of falls and fractures. Yet, if we are at all able to move, we can do much to prevent muscle atrophy by incorporating the *Reclaim 24* Workout.

Researchers have found that muscle atrophy resulting from long periods of inactivity or immobility is hard for older people to overcome. If they kick off an exercise program with too much intensity, they may generate scar tissue, inflammation, and unusual soreness instead of muscle—effects that younger people don't experience. So it's important to start slowly and gently, working at a pace that fits your age and current level of fitness. I believe it's never too late to begin an exercise regimen, but you must be sensible in your approach, especially if you are older. Get professional help from a properly educated personal trainer or physical therapist. That's the wise and safe way to go, especially if you are new to exercise or you have not exercised in a while.

New research is beginning to show why aging muscles don't respond to exercise as well as younger muscles. It was already known that older people don't use ingested protein as well as younger people to make muscle. Now they've also found[7] that insulin released during meals does not work as well with older people as with younger. With younger folks, released insulin suppresses the metabolic breakdown of muscle (for fuel) during "fasting" periods (overnight and between meals). But for older people, insulin *does not* suppress muscle breakdown quite as well. The researchers also found that the blood flow to older muscles is less than that to the muscles of younger people. That got them asking: "Does muscle wasting in older people occur because decreased blood flow reduces the supply of hormones (insulin) and protein to those muscles?"

Exercise, they reasoned, is a natural remedy for poor blood circulation. So, in the study, they followed up with the older group by having them take three weight-training sessions per week over 20 weeks. From this the research team confirmed that the exercise regimen rejuvenated blood flow in the extremities of the older group *to the point where it was identical to that of the younger group!*

---

7 Eurekalert, "Muscle: 'Hard to build, easy to lose' as you age,"
Nottingham University, September 11, 2009.

Does this experimental result confirm that exercise may protect muscles from wasting away in older people? We will have to wait for further confirmation, but the research findings so far seem to be saying, "use it or lose it."

Yes, as we age, physical exercise becomes ever more important for retaining optimal health. Even longevity. Nature has programmed the human body to enter decline after the procreation years of the teens, 20's, and early 30's. This natural decline with age (stress buildup) can be seen in all organ and hormonal systems of the body. But as humans, we can forestall these natural tendencies for many decades by changing the way we do things—*by changing our habits to reduce stress and to support our stress-fighting biological functions.* The problem is that most people want to follow the "path of least resistance" (an apt phrase in this chapter) and hope that nature will continue to support them as it did in their procreation years. But it will not—at least not without help.

My 67-year-old editor relates that when he was 43—he remembers it well—he would come home after a full day's work and sit on his couch exhausted. It felt so darn good not to move! It was the *natural* thing to do. Yet, his couch time seemed to replenish his energy stores less and less over time. He knew he was losing something.

Then one evening as he sat there, he had an epiphany of sorts. He realized that he was carving a future pathway towards even further inactivity and physical decline. The handwriting on the wall was suddenly clear! At that moment, he decided he wasn't going to take the "natural," lazy route any longer. He was going to start *moving* just as he had in his teens, 20's, and 30's. It didn't make any difference that his peers weren't moving; he would. So he went out for a labored jog but was nonetheless energized from the effort. An oxygen infusion!

A week later, he bought a cheap weight bench and weights to take care of the resistance training side of his epiphany. That was the turning point—the beginning of the rest of his self-care life. He wasn't going to follow the path of least resistance because he could clearly see where it was leading—the Pits of Despair—and he didn't want to go there!

Since then he has embraced many wellness opportunities to challenge the natural decline that accompanies the path of least resistance. He says he's glad he has done so. It's been a worthwhile investment of time, effort, and money for him. But there had to be an investment. Nature doesn't hand out gifts.

So let's take this idea a step further. Many common diseases spring from a sedentary lifestyle such as diabetes, heart disease, and osteoporosis. In addition, limited ranges of motion, aches and pains, and excessive muscle wasting also arise. Under these conditions, resistance training is probably your answer for maintaining optimal health well into your senior years.

How Resistance Training Can Reduce Your Disease Risks (e.g., Diabetes, Heart Disease, and Dangerous Organ Fat)

Your body has two types of fat: visceral and subcutaneous. Subcutaneous fat is located just below your skin and is the type that causes dimpling and cellulite. Visceral fat, on the other hand, shows up in your abdomen and surrounds your vital organs including your liver, heart, and muscles. It is visceral fat that has been linked to serious health problems such as heart disease, diabetes, stroke, insulin resistance, and many other chronic diseases or problems.

We've learned that a key strategy for reducing your risk of heart disease and a host of other chronic diseases is to keep your systemic inflammation levels low. Another key strategy is to avoid gaining visceral fat in the first place—or to reduce what's already there. Exercise—especially resistance training because of its effect on muscle development—offers a double-barreled solution. It both lowers hidden inflammation in your body and is one of the best weapons against visceral fat. For example, in one study,[8] volunteers who did not exercise had an 8.6 percent increase in visceral fat after eight months, while those who exercised the most lost over 8 percent of their visceral fat during the same period.

As I emphasized in earlier chapters, muscle tissue burns many calories not only when it is in use but also when at rest. Yes, muscle tissue is metabolically active around the clock, even when you're sleeping. It's your 24/7 solution to burning calories! So, as you gain muscle, your body naturally increases the amount of calories burned each day. This reduces fat stores if your hormone system is working properly.

As for lowering inflammation, physical exercise accomplishes this naturally by lowering levels of a C-reactive protein (CRP), a blood

---

[8] *ScienceDaily*, May 29, 2003.

protein linked to hidden inflammation. High levels of CRP in your body are associated with a higher than average risk of cardiovascular disease. These days, CRP levels are better indicators of heart attack risk than high cholesterol. In fact, you'll be hearing less and less about cholesterol with time because the cholesterol myth is being busted. But Big Pharma will keep the home fires burning as long as possible in order to sell cholesterol-lowering drugs. So ...

Beware of Drugs that Can Cause Irreversible Damage to Your Muscles

Aside from a sedentary lifestyle, another common cause of excessive muscle wasting is the use of statins, a class of cholesterol-lowering drugs with many dangerous side effects. Statins such as Lipitor, Zocor, Pavacol and Mevacor lower your cholesterol by inhibiting HMG-CoA reductase, a key enzyme in cholesterol synthesis. But they can also activate the atrogin-1 gene. That gene plays a key role in muscle atrophy. A recent study[9] showed that even low concentrations of statins lead to atrogin-1-induced muscle damage. And the higher the dosage, the greater the damage. Since your heart is a muscle, this side effect can lead to quite unpleasant side effects!

The moral? Practice wellness so you don't have to get into trouble in the first place.

How Strength Training Reduces Osteoporosis

Weight-bearing exercise is one of the most effective remedies against osteoporosis. Taking drugs is the last thing you want to do to improve your bone density. Without question, bone-density drugs are more likely to cause long-term harm than bring benefits. These drugs do indeed make your bones more dense, as the drug commercials suggest, but *not* stronger—which the drug commercials *do not suggest*! How can that be? Imagine a glass tube. Fill it with sand to increase the density. Will that make the tube stronger and prevent it from breaking?

Your bones are actually porous and soft. As you get older, they can easily become less dense and consequently more brittle, especially if you are inactive. Resistance training can counter this effect if your nutrition and hormone balances are right. As you put more tension on your

---

[9] *The Journal of Clinical Investigation,* Dec 2007; 117(12):3940-51.

muscles, it puts more pressure on your bones, which then respond by continuously creating fresh, new bone (which the drugs don't do). Also, as you build more muscle and strengthen the muscles that you already have, muscle tone itself puts more pressure on your bones, *constantly.* This constant stress induces bone strengthening.

Do Keep Yourself in Motion!

I can say one thing with confidence: I've had considerable experience with older patients, associates, and friends who train with resistance and who have adopted a wellness lifestyle. That experience tells me that it has worked wonders for them. I'm confident future research will continue to confirm what I already know about the wellness lifestyle for older people. But it's important for you to understand that the earlier you adopt a *Reclaim 24* lifestyle, the more value you will get from it. The declines that come from inactivity, or from other poor health habits, build up over time and are seldom fully reversible.

Optimal health is dependent on an active lifestyle in addition to other wellness-practice behaviors listed on page 25. So start moving—and don't stop no matter what your age! If you do stop, you'll find that nature has reserved a seat for you—or a bed, as the case may be—on that infamous Conveyor Belt to a Living Hell.

And do follow the *Reclaim 24* resistance-training regimen unless your physical condition precludes it. The *Reclaim 24* Workout is the number one way for you to remain strong, young, and independent—well into advanced age.

Now, let's jump into the fitness part of your 12-week action plan: the *Reclaim 24* Workout.

8: The *Reclaim 24* Workout Explained

Y ou'll need only 24 hours of actual fitness training to achieve a welcome and easily recognized body metamorphosis. I've structured my program so you make these changes over a 12-week period, meaning you perform no more than two—2—hours of total exercise each week. I'll repeat that again: TWO HOURS PER WEEK.

The workout is divided into three different sessions per week, always with one or two days of rest between sessions (including one or two days of rest between the last session of one week and the first session of the next). These three weekly sessions are your *push day*, your *pull day*, and your *legs day*. You devote each session to muscle groups or body parts as described next.

Your Three Weekly Sessions

- On your PUSH DAY, you exercise: *Chest, Shoulders, Triceps*
- On your PULL DAY, you exercise: *Back, Biceps, Abdominals*
- On your LEGS DAY, you exercise: *Quadriceps, Hamstrings, Calves*

On each of the three days, you perform two exercises per body part, such as your chest. And you perform each exercise over two sets. For example, on your push day, the following *preliminary* table applies—which doesn't include warm-up sets yet:

PUSH DAY	EXERCISE	SETS TO FAILURE
Chest	Upright Chest Press	2
	Flat Bench Flyes	2
Shoulders	Seated Dumbbell Press	2
	Standing Dumbbell Laterals	2
Triceps	Close-Grip Pushdown	2
	Lying Triceps Press	2

The table shows that you perform two different exercises for your chest, two for your shoulders, and two for your triceps. Further, each of the six exercises must be done twice—two sets per exercise (I'll explain "sets to failure" in a little bit). Don't worry if you don't know what the exercise names mean. That information is available in Appendix A with photos and plenty of explanation on how to perform the exercises.

If you do your arithmetic right, you'll see that for each workout day, you'll perform exactly 12 sets, with four sets dedicated to each body part or muscle group for that day. In a little bit, you'll see that you also need to include warm-up sets.

To avoid boredom, and to keep your muscles from adapting and becoming too "efficient" for effective growth, you want to avoid performing the <u>same exercise</u> more than once for the given body part during that day's workout (which would amount to all four sets using the same equipment and same motion). Rather, you want to choose two *different* exercises from a menu of exercises for that body part. This gives your muscles some variety.

As the table shows, to train your chest muscles on your push day, you might choose to do two sets of the "upright chest press" on a machine designed for upright presses and two sets on a flat bench with an exercise called a "flat bench fly." In Appendix A, I've illustrated sample exercises that you can use for this program, along with explanations of how to perform them. To watch videos of how to perform those and other exercises, please visit my website, **www.drcharleswebb.com.** There you'll also find photos and explanations for additional exercise options that you may want to use for variety in your workouts.

So, once you've performed your four sets for each body part or muscle group, you're done for the day! Then, except perhaps for some social time with others in the gym, you head for home.

What "Sets to Failure" Means

Now, I'll explain what I mean by "sets to failure." <u>This is the key for transforming your body in 24 hour's worth of exercise</u>. Each of the 12 sets[10] must be done until the muscle(s) you're training become exhausted! In body-shaping lingo, we call this "training the muscle to failure." So you're not just counting some fixed number of repetitions and then stopping. You're pushing your muscles hard enough to reach the point where you simply CANNOT do one more complete repetition

---

[10] In this chapter, I recommend you perform *two* sets to muscle failure for each different exercise. If you are *truly* capable of performing sets to failure—and most people don't get very close to it without introductory training from a professional—then you can get fine results by performing just one failure set per exercise for a total of six. This shortens your workout even further, but it does require focus and dedication. And warmups are still essential.

or movement! *That's* when the set is over (and <u>not</u> after you've counted 10 repetitions, for example).

This means if you initially planned a ballpark number of 10 repetitions in a set, you don't stop at 10 just because you've reached it. Instead, you must push and push, adding further repetitions until your muscles fail you (whether it's more or less than the ballpark 10). Remember, your muscles will not grow well with low-intensity exercises. You need to place the most stress on them that you can. I'll talk more about this in the upcoming section, *Exercise Quality Is Crucial*.

Warmups Are Essential

If you've done any weight training before, you might now be asking about the need to warm up before attempting your failure sets. And you'd be right to ask! Yes, indeed, <u>you do need to include warmup sets prior to the intense sets shown in the above table</u>. So the first table must be augmented just a bit. What follows is what the final push-day table looks like after we add warmups (and totals) to the picture.

Push Day

PUSH DAY	EXERCISE	WARMUP SETS	SETS TO FAILURE
Chest	Upright Chest Press	2	2
	Flat bench Flyes	1	2
Shoulders	Seated Dumbbell Press	1	2
	Standing Dumbbell Laterals	0	2
Triceps	Close-Grip Pushdowns	1	2
	Lying Triceps Press	0	2
Totals		5	12

You always need a couple of warmup sets to start your exercise routine for the session because your muscles are cold and unprepared. Cold muscles simply won't work as well as those that you've warmed up, and you won't be able to get the greatest benefit from your routine. Furthermore, a cold muscle is *much* more prone to injury, and injury is not a designated part of my wellness program! Warmups get the blood flowing in the muscles for better nutrient support and waste removal. They also kick off the process of "neuromuscular recruitment," which means that your brain and nervous system are starting to gear up for the tasks to come. (I'll explain *neuromuscular recruitment* in more detail at the end of this chapter.)

This final table considers several points. For one thing, both warm-up and high-intensity sets have "carry-over" value for later sets so that you have to execute fewer warmup sets. This is so because some muscle groups are warmed up to a certain degree with each exercise, and the need to perform the same level of warmup for succeeding exercises goes away. Nevertheless, to avoid injury and to properly activate neuromuscular recruitment, a single warmup set is *always* warranted when beginning a new muscle group.

How to Perform Warmup Sets. *You don't perform warmup sets to failure,* or even to any great level of intensity. Nor should they exceed about eight repetitions for the set (an eight count is okay for warmups).

When performing warmup sets, you want to use a weight that is about 70%-80% of the weight you plan to use in the intense sets. You need not perform more than 6-8 repetitions for a warm-up set to be effective.

Can you see now that your total time in the gym is not going to be that great? With this program, you do not spend more than 30 minutes total time performing resistance exercises. If you perform these sets correctly, you have no need for additional sets. In fact, doing additional sets can be counterproductive because they may result in overtraining.

If you are new to resistance training, or you don't have the slightest idea what kinds of resistances to start with, make sure you consult a professional to get you started.

Some people simply cannot handle much resistance at all because their current organ and glandular condition worsens with the additional stress of high-intensity physical activity. They may easily tire during warmups or even find themselves feeling worse for a day or more after a workout (but simple muscle soreness doesn't count as "worse" because it's actually better). Such people *must* work with both a professional at the gym and a wellness doctor who can keep them from going places they shouldn't. Remember this: under your wellness practice, 5% or more of it is devoted to handling conditions or situations that may not respond well to self-care. So professional help is in order.

* * *

Your "Pull Day" and "Legs Day" are designed the same way as your "Push Day." Here are example workout tables for these two days (you may choose different exercises for each body part as shown in Appendix A and on my website at **www.drcharleswebb.com**).

Pull Day

PULL DAY	EXERCISE	WARMUPS SETS	SETS TO FAILURE
Back	Wide Grip Pull-Downs	2	2
	One-Arm Dumbbell Rows	1	2
Biceps	Standing Dumbbell Curls	1	2
	Preacher Curls	0	2
Abdominals	Twist Crunches	1	2
	Pelvic Roll-Ups	0	2
Totals		5	12

Legs Day

LEGS DAY	EXERCISE	WARMUP SETS	SETS TO FAILURE
Quadriceps	Leg Press	2	2
	Leg Extensions	1	2
Hamstrings	Lying Leg Curls	1	2
	Dumbbell Lunges	0	2
Calves	Seated Calf Raises	1	2
	One-Legged Calf Raise	0	2
Totals		5	12

Exercise Quality Is Crucial

How you perform your individual sets is just as important as the intensity. In fact, it's the key to being able to place the maximum amount of stress on muscles without having to use a substantial amount of weight or risk injury.

Muscles are made up of bundles of fibers that contract. Individual fibers within these bundles react in "all or nothing" patterns. In other words, any given fiber—called a myofibril—is either fully "fired" by the nervous system for shortening, or it isn't fired at all. This means that the variability in contraction of the *overall* muscle is based on the *number* of fibers that contract. Therefore, good muscle-building exercises engage as many muscle fibers as possible and for a sufficient amount of time to stimulate them fully. Muscles grow best with such intense stimulation.

Overcoming the Instinct to "Make Things Easy"

One of the greatest handicaps an undisciplined body builder or body shaper faces is the strong impulse to perform any given exercise *in the easiest way possible*. This means he or she instinctively takes advantage of inertia and the ready "availability" of adjoining muscles (plus posture deviations) to complete a given repetition. This is called "cheating" in gym parlance, and the impulse must be replaced with something better.

For example, when doing a standing biceps curl, if the beginning of the movement is used to start the weight into a "swing" motion, then the lifter is able to reduce the amount of effort required during the last part of the upward movement because the weight has been "launched," so to speak.

The problem with cheating is that fewer muscle fibers are stimulated to contract than if a slower, more controlled approach is used to lift the weight. In other words, for muscle building, well-controlled movements do not use inertia to aid completion. Remember, the name of the game is to stimulate as many fibers as possible, *but only in the muscle group being trained*. Inertial movements and other forms of cheating work against this. That's why my program avoids such movements.

The common problem with inertial movements is they usually require the assistance of other muscle groups in order to gather the momentum needed for cheating. These are muscles that you *don't* want to train with the given exercise. For example, it's common to see a lifter arch his or her back during the explosive part of a biceps curl. This certainly makes the curl easier. But it defeats the principle of maximum muscle-fiber stimulation. The result is that the bicep group you *want* to train isn't getting its fully intended benefit because other muscle groups—in both the back and the shoulders—have inadvertently been recruited during the

78

movement to make the biceps curl easier. So, fewer bicep muscle fibers get stimulated. See?

The solution to the problem of inertia and cheating is to attempt to complete your repetition in a slow and controlled manner while staunchly retaining your posture. In this way, you stress the largest number of fibers in the desired muscle group. This stimulates the muscle group to its full capacity.

To perform your repetitions in a slow, controlled, posture-preserving manner may mean you have to use a lighter weight initially. As you continue to exercise properly, you soon find your strength increasing. Along with this, the need to increase the weight.

How slowly should you perform a repetition? Let me give you my experience. Over the years I've experimented with the explosive rep as well as the slow rep and have found that as long as I am controlling the movement, the speed is probably right. However, as I've aged, it's become less desirable and more uncomfortable to train with excessively heavy weight. So, I've chosen to work out with more moderate weights. By slowing down my repetitions to a three-to-four second cadence in both the contracting direction and relaxing direction, I've still been able to provide an optimal amount of muscle stress while using less weight. And so the muscle growth and maintenance continues. This slower movement also puts less stress on my joints and tendons.

The Two Phases of Contraction

Resistance training requires opposite movements for each exercise repetition. The first part of the movement, Phase 1, contracts the muscles being stimulated, which means tightening and shortening. Phase 2, the second part of the movement, reverses the effect of Phase 1. This means Phase 2 relaxes and lengthens the muscles being trained so you can get back to your original position. For the best results, *both* phases should be done slowly and in a controlled way, not just Phase 1. And keep in mind that both phases require some level of muscle contraction. It's just that Phase 2 reduces the intensity of contraction enough so that the machine or weight resistance takes you back to your starting point so you can repeat Phase 1.

For example, raising a weight with a biceps curl tightens and shortens the biceps, while lowering the weight back to its original position lengthens the biceps. Pressing a barbell upward during a bench press tightens and shortens the triceps, and letting the weight return to your chest in a slow release relaxes and lengthens the triceps.

Numerous studies have shown that slow, controlled movements in *both* directions are necessary to stimulate a muscle to its full capacity. That's why it's so important to move through an *entire* repetition slowly and deliberately (except for *partial reps,* to be discussed in a minute). You should know, however, that certain pieces of hydraulic equipment now being used in some ladies' gyms only support the contraction or muscle-shortening phase of an exercise, ultimately limiting the overall progress and muscle development of those who use that equipment.

How to Achieve "Intensity"

I explained the importance of high-intensity training earlier, but how do you achieve this? Well, one component of intensity is making certain you continue to push through your set until your muscles can no longer complete a full additional repetition. This is what we call "proceeding to muscle failure." This means that, on a scale of 1 to 10, *you should be performing at intensity level 10 for each set that isn't a warm-up set.* It's because of this 10-level intensity that only four total sets are needed to maximize the stress load on the muscle or muscle group you're training. Besides, after pushing this hard for four sets, you won't want to do additional sets!

To enhance high-intensity training even further, we use techniques to stress muscles at the end of a set, *after* you've completed your final full repetition. These techniques add to the intensity level, which in turn force the muscle to continue to respond and develop. I like to use three different techniques for achieving this: partial reps, drop sets, and "forced" reps. Forced reps require a "spotter" or training partner, while a spotter is optional for partial reps and drop sets. Here's how these techniques work.

Partial Reps

Partial repetitions are self-descriptive. When you're convinced you are in the midst of the very last complete rep that you can eke out in your current set, and you're under the full Phase 1 contraction for that final rep, then don't allow the muscle to fully release in Phase 2; *just release part way.* Then start a full Phase 1 contraction again! It's sort of a mini rep in which you don't use the full range of motion that otherwise might be available to you. Though you probably couldn't have done another full rep, you usually can squeeze a partial rep or two out of your exhausted muscles.

For example, if you're performing your "final" bench press rep for a set, the full Phase 1 contraction occurs when you press the weight furthest away from your body with your arms fully extended. From this position, you allow the weight to come toward you only part way before pressing it to the full, extended position once again.

I recommend that you perform partials with a partner (spotter) standing by to help you. The exception is for exercises that don't put you at risk if you should fail during a full or partial rep. For example, performing "Pull" exercises such as the Lat Pull Down or Biceps Curl generally doesn't pose any threat and you don't need a spotter to protect you if you fail. If you're using a machine instead of free weights, you can also avoid the need of a partner or spotter since the machine won't collapse on you. I often prefer machines to free weights for that very reason. They allow me to push to the optimum point of failure without worrying about finishing the rep or injuring myself.

When choosing the partial rep technique at the end of a set, you only need to perform two partial repetitions. To avoid overtraining, this technique should be used only with the *second* high-intensity set performed for each exercise. Don't use it with the first set.

The "Drop Set"

This technique works quite well, especially if you prefer free weights or don't have access to machines. The "Drop Set" implies dropping down to a lighter weight to accomplish an additional two or three repetitions once you've reached muscle failure in the primary set. For example, assume you've just completed your second set of dumbbell shoulder presses to the point of failure. You know you cannot possibly perform another repetition on your own. So you now place the dumbbells on the floor and quickly grab a *lighter* set that allows you to perform a few extra repetitions. Don't take any more time than necessary for exchanging weights before continuing the set. This technique works well with both machines and weights and doesn't require that you use a spotter.

Forced Reps Plus "Spotter"

When you are near the end of a set and your muscles become just too exhausted to complete even one more full rep with good form, you may eke out a few more <u>forced reps</u> with the help of a spotter. A "spotter" is a workout partner or trainer who helps you complete your sets. When you are doing forced reps, this person physically helps you move the weight through the entire starting and finishing ranges of motion because you can't do it on your own.

As with partial reps, you should restrict forced reps to two or three additional movements. And, as with partial reps, <u>forced reps should only be used on the last set</u> of each high-intensity exercise.

Many people find that having a workout partner motivates them and pushes them beyond what they normally would ask of themselves. For this reason alone I highly recommend finding someone with whom you are likely to be compatible. Please use caution here. If your partner isn't as motivated as you and consistently misses workouts or is frequently late, look for another. Half-motivated "partners" only limit your progress.

How Many Repetitions Get the Best Results?

To repeat, more important than the number of repetitions in a set is the *quality and intensity of the movements you perform.* The most crucial set in any given workout is the one you're performing *now*, meaning not the last one you did or the next one, but *this* one. Always concentrate solely on your current set and finish it with your best effort. With that said, let's talk about reps.

All in all, a rep range between 6 and 12 allows you to adequately stimulate the most fibers and therefore best stimulate muscle growth. For beginners I recommend initially choosing resistances or weights that keep you around the 10–12 repetition range. Later, attempt heavier weight that force you into the 6-8 rep range. But please don't preoccupy yourself with the number of repetitions completed as long as you can feel you're taxing your muscles to their limits. Personally, I often alter the weight I use to keep a muscle group from adapting to my workouts. Of course, the rep ranges must also change to accommodate the different weights.

82

One more thing. You'll no doubt hear, if you haven't already, that repetitions in the range of 15 to 20 are better when trying to achieve greater muscle definition. This is ludicrous. You get lean when you add muscle and watch your diet, not when you simply perform many repetitions in a set. If you want to do 15 to 20 reps for the occasional "shock value" to your muscles to help prevent adaptation, go ahead. Just don't feel that you need to do it often or that it will help you get the definition you seek. It won't.

Rest Periods: How Many? How Long?

How much rest should you allow between sets? As a rule of thumb, you need only 30 seconds of rest following warm-up sets and about 60 seconds between your high-intensity sets. The main point is to make certain you have ample time to recuperate between your high-intensity sets. A little more or less than 60 seconds isn't going to make a difference.

The actual time it takes to complete a set should be about 45-60 seconds, give or take a few seconds. So adding up the total time of the resistance training session, we get the following:

- 5 total warm-up sets at 40 seconds = 3.5 minutes

- 5 rest periods at 30 seconds = 2.5 minutes

- 12 total intensity sets at 60 seconds = 12 minutes

- 12 rest periods at 60 seconds = 12 minutes

Total workout time = 30 minutes

Note: You may use your rest periods to move to different pieces of equipment, change weights, or re-hydrate.

The Role Played by "Neuromuscular Recruitment"

This term is really less technical than it sounds at first blush. It makes sense with a simple explanation.

For a muscle to contract, there must be a signal sent from your brain to activate the fibers that make up the bulk of that muscle. When preparing to lift a pencil, your brain sends signals to just enough fibers to accomplish this task (remember, the fibers that make up a muscle contract independently and are either contracted completely or not contracted at all). Because you've trained your brain to know that the weight of a pencil is quite small, the proper signals are sent to the muscles of your arm, hand, and fingers to fire the minimal number of fibers to get the expected job done.

Now, let's suppose you're instructed to bend down and lift a barbell weighing 200 lbs. Knowing this, you prepare yourself mentally, get into position, breathe in deeply, and go for it. But what if someone has fooled you and the real weight of the barbell is only 10 lbs? What will happen? You will most likely jerk that weight with everything you have and fall on your backside in total surprise.

That's neuromuscular recruitment in action! Your nervous system recruits the number of muscle fibers it *expects* will be required for the task at hand. In the above situation, your brain is fooled into thinking it needs to send enough signals to your muscles to achieve a 200 lbs. lift when in fact the weight is only 10 lbs. Because of this, *all* your muscle fibers contract. But when it turns out the actual resistance is only 10 lbs, you fall on your butt. On the other hand, if you know beforehand that the weight is only 10 lbs., your nervous system does the right thing and you complete your lift eloquently (we can hope).

When it comes to resistance training, it's important to condition your brain to effectively and efficiently do its job. Your warm-up sets not only warm your muscles for the more intense sets to come but also "remind" the brain that more weight is on the way and that the right amount of neuromuscular recruitment must take place to handle the greater stress. The brain therefore prepares itself to send out the number of signals needed for you to lift the heaviest weight you can for 6–12 intense reps. Furthermore, two intense sets per exercise rather than one convinces the brain to activate greater numbers of fibers. Therefore, you get better "coverage."

9: The Truth about Cardiovascular Training

True aerobic training calls for raising the heart rate into an acceptable range, which is dependent on age, in order to burn fat for energy. Do you accept that?

I don't know who conducted the research studies that determined the generally acceptable heart-rate ranges for age groups. Nor do I know how they performed the research. I'm definitely more fit than the majority of men at my age of 49. Yet, according to the chart on the stair-stepper at my gym, I should keep my heart rate between 120-130 beats per minute. But when I work in that range, I exert little effort. Why should I restrict myself to what the chart says if it's only judging my health by my age? And why shouldn't I follow the guidelines for men in the 30-35 year range if that coincides more closely with my fitness level? I certainly feel I can keep up with them.

I ask these rhetorical questions to point out that the information you get regarding cardiovascular training may be as much myth as science. Moreover, the pervasive myth seriously overestimates the ability of cardio to shed fat and chisel the abs. Therefore, you can relax if you thought I was going to tell you that you must do 30-40 minutes of aerobic training five days a week. That's enough to scare most people to the couch. It's true that maintaining your heart rate at an elevated but not an overly rapid rate for a period of 15 minutes or more coaxes your metabolism into shifting gears to burn fat as its main fuel source. Isn't this what everyone wants? Of course it is, but there are different ways to meet this goal—some better than others.

Aerobics, Alone, Won't Give You the Shape You Want!

If you've ever tried to lose weight and tone up through aerobics, whether on a stationary bike or a treadmill or by attending aerobics classes, you probably weren't overly impressed with your results. Granted, if you increase your energy expenditure while keeping your calories the same, you eventually lose some weight. But did the shape of your new body look much different from when you started? Did you really see those muscles taking on a distinct shape and firmness? Heck, did you see any muscles at all?

Don't feel bad. You're not the only one who's spent persistent, boring hours on cardio equipment trying to burn off that large dinner from the night before. And by the way, something else happens when you begin to do a lot of aerobic training. Your appetite grows. This typically leads to a vicious cycle as you try to do even more aerobics to burn more calories and then eat more to feed your body's increased demand for fuel. This is a cycle not worth starting. My point is this:

> ## Aerobic training has little if any effect on changing the shape of your body.

If you're lucky, you may actually lose some weight over time. But then you just become a flabby skinny person. Why, then, do all the so-called fitness "gurus" say you must do aerobic training?

Because they are working with the wrong information.

The truth is, I don't at all feel guilty about coaxing people away from spending hours per week on bikes or treadmills or jogging if what they really want is a better toned and shaped body! So let's look at the facts.

When you exercise in the aerobic range, you burn about 120-150 calories every 20 minutes, depending on your size and fitness level. If you do this three times a week, every week, you burn about 1,620 additional calories for the month. Whoopee!

Now here's an interesting point. For every pound of muscle you develop, your body burns over 1,500 calories per month just to maintain it. The fact is, muscles are calorie-burning machines—not only during exercise but also at rest! Further, when you keep your insulin[11] levels at the lower end of the health range during both aerobic exercise periods and during rest periods (which are also aerobic), your body automatically dives into your fat reserves for energy.

So if you were to put on an additional two pounds of muscle, that extra muscle would automatically burn up more than 3,000 calories per month—*the equivalent of about 5, 20-minute aerobic sessions per week!* Now can you see why developing muscle is so valuable for weight control? It takes a lot of caloric energy to build *and maintain* lean tissue, whereas fat barely requires any energy at all to maintain. In fact, fat *is* energy in potential form—pure fuel stored away in globs around your body.

---

[11] More about the effect of insulin in Chapter 10, "Rejuvenate with Nourishment."

Therefore, if you want to change your body composition, waste no more of your precious time trying to do it with boring aerobic activities. Too much aerobic training can actually hinder your progress since it can lead both to muscle atrophy and a slower metabolism. However, if you feel you really want to take part in an occasional aerobics class, spin class, or romp on the treadmill or stair-stepper, go for it. But do it for the fun of it as well as the cardiovascular fitness. Just limit such activities to two or three sessions per week. Although jogging on a treadmill won't offer much in the way of toning and shaping your body, it offers tremendous benefits toward your cardiovascular health.

My 12-week *Reclaim 24* Action Plan advocates replacing regular aerobic activities with moderately paced resistance training plus high-intensity interval training. Each of these replacements helps you develop cardiovascular fitness as well as reshape your body. If you choose not to follow my type of fitness program, you need to do the boring stuff to retain cardiovascular health. And you may be destined to remain a flabby skinny person.

The Advantages of High-Intensity Interval Training

Although I don't see much value in low-intensity aerobic training for body shaping, I do know it's important to maintain cardiovascular fitness. Any type of exercise that makes the heart and lungs work harder is, by definition, cardiovascular fitness training. This includes moderately paced resistance training. As you move through your *Reclaim 24* Workout, you soon find you have no time to chat with fellow gym members or take calls on your cell phone. Instead, you have to focus and move through the workout at a steady pace if you are to complete it in the allotted 30 minutes. This keeps your heart rate elevated throughout the session and improves your cardiovascular fitness as a result. But for those of you who wish to really get the heart and lungs pumping, I've included 10 minutes of interval training *at the end of your resistance training*.

Cardiovascular interval training is a high-intensity, short-duration type of exertion meant to work the heart and lungs as well as burn off excessive glycogen stores. The burn-off works like this...

The blood sugar, glucose, is stored within the muscles or liver as glycogen, a form of animal starch that the body quickly and easily converts back to glucose. The interesting thing about glucose is that it requires no oxygen to burn. This means it is an anaerobic fuel ideal for supplying energy bursts during high-intensity, short-duration workouts where oxygen is in short supply. However, here's where things get dicey. The brain runs on glucose and protects itself more than any other organ. After all, it is the body's command and control center. Therefore, when glycogen stores start running low, the brain conserves a quantity for its own use and automatically shifts to other sources of fuel to support the body's energy needs. In fact, the brain signals the body to cannibalize its own lean tissue and stored fat, converting them to glucose and certain types of fatty acids that will burn for fuel. Your lean tissue, by the way, includes muscle, bone, and connective tissue—none of which you want to be using for fuel!

However, fat converts more slowly to fuel than does muscle, bone, and connective tissue. This means that under *anaerobic* conditions, where the largest amounts of energy are needed in a short period, fat is the last source to be used for fuel. So, any time your workout uses up too much glycogen, you are putting your muscles and other lean tissue at risk of being used for fuel. This is the last thing you want your workouts to do for you!

However, once an intense workout has ended and you are back in an *aerobic* state, the body's demand for quick energy lessens. In its biological wisdom, the body happily switches to metabolizing stored fat for fuel rather than consume its lean tissue. Fat's slower conversion rate doesn't serve as a hindrance under these conditions because the rate is sufficient to meet the lower energy needs. And your fat reserves *will* burn if your hormone system, including your leptin metabolism, is healthy.

So, the secret is to keep your workout short and sweet. You burn up much of your glycogen stores during the 30 minutes of high-intensity resistance training and consume an additional amount during your 10-minute interval training that immediately follows. With your 40-minute high-intensity-plus-interval-training workout, you deplete a large portion of your body's glycogen stores *without getting into the danger zone*. Then, when your workout has ended, the brain knows it's safe to shift more fully into using the body's fat reserves for fuel.

In fact, you want to take advantage of the brain's fat-burning process following your workout. *This means ingesting nothing but water until your body gives you a hunger signal.* That hunger signal may arrive in five minutes after you finish (not typical at all), or maybe a couple of hours after you finish. Before the hunger signal arrives, you will have a clear head and a feeling of good energy that follows healthy workouts.

When the hunger signal does arrive, it means your brain no longer wants to burn the fatty acids that have been released into the bloodstream and instead wants to replenish your exercised muscles and other tissues for growth and recuperation. But there's more. Because of how your leptin metabolism works, your muscle building *efficiency* is the highest of all when you postpone eating until you are actually hungry! Further, you get the most fat-burning benefit when exercising at least three or more hours *after* a meal. Combine these two principles and you can nicely link fat burning and muscle building by timing your exercise routines to closely precede mealtimes. Of course, *for some people* this means less energy being available for challenging workout routines. Such individuals do better eating something an hour or two before exercise. So each of us needs to feel our way to our best exercise times. Often, life doesn't give us much of a detailed choice and we exercise when we can find the time!

But please take note: once the hunger signal arrives following exercise, you don't want to postpone eating for very long—no more than 30 to 45 minutes. Why? Because if you don't satisfy the hunger signal in less than an hour of its receipt, your brain will shut your metabolism way down and at the same time set up lengthy cravings out of fear of starvation. You may actually end up gaining weight in the next day or so. I'm sure you have experienced getting "over hungry" from missing a meal and seeing how hard it is to satisfy your appetite once that happens.

By using my exercise strategy, you not only exercise your heart and lungs, but you also get a period of fat burning (5 minutes to 2 hours or more) during the rest period before your next meal. Doesn't this sound like a better alternative to your typical aerobic workout?

Now, most people don't know this, but interval training—which means go fast then go slow then repeat—offers definite advantages over low-intensity cardio work, even though it is more challenging. For example:

1. It burns more calories than low-intensity training, meaning you can burn more fat in shorter workouts if you do it right.

2. Higher intensities stimulate your metabolism far more *after* the workout ends than lower intensities do. This means you continue to burn calories and fat for long periods after you finish training.

This is not true with low-intensity training, where the elevated calorie burn rate drops close to normal when you are finished.

3. As with training at high intensity, training at higher speeds can dramatically improve sports performance for those interested in such achievements. Football players can sprint faster and recover more quickly between plays. Tennis players can keep chasing down balls during longer points. Even endurance athletes benefit by conditioning their bodies to work at a faster pace.

And so, that's why 10 minutes of high-intensity interval training is a part of the *Reclaim 24* System.

To perform the interval training exercise, you need to find a piece of cardio equipment you're comfortable with, be it a treadmill, elliptical trainer, or stair stepper. If you enjoy the outdoors, you can perform this type of training with a bike or even on foot. The idea is to elevate your heart rate by **aggressively pumping your legs** for one-minute intervals while moving at a more moderate pace between the intense intervals. Your intensity level should allow you to push through an entire 60 seconds, but not much longer. If you find you're able to move at your "intense" pace for more than two minutes, you need to up your intensity level or resistance setting on the machine. As you complete each one-minute interval, you lower your intensity or setting to allow yourself to catch your breath.

Let's assume you've chosen the stair stepper to perform your exercise. By trial and error, you soon learn, for example, that a level-12 setting on the machine creates high intensity for you. Your workout would look something like this, assuming the example of level 12 being your high-intensity setting:

STAIR STEPPER (Total Time = 10 Minutes)
- 2 minutes on level 6 to warm-up
- 1 minute on level 12
- 1 minute on level 8
- 1 minute on level 12
- 1 minute on level 8
- 1 minute on level 12
- 1 minute on level 8
- 1 minute on level 12
- 1 minute on level 8 (Follow with 1-2 minute cool down)

So there you have it. The total time for the entire workout is 40 minutes (30 minutes of resistance training and another 10 minutes of high-intensity interval training). This is all the time you need to develop the body of your dreams. If your fitness goals are moderate, you may even do less, but follow the same principles.

As an example of a more moderate approach, you may want to start out by performing only one exercise per body part, which cuts your workout down to 25 minutes. If you're resting properly and eating right, you'll still see dramatic results even with this less-aggressive approach. Whatever approach you choose, however, make it your personal decision, one that you're comfortable with and *one that you know you can stick with.*

I would like to reemphasize that before beginning the high-intensity workout and interval training outlined in this book, I recommend you visit your doctor if you have any health concerns. Such concerns would include, but not be limited to, high blood pressure, obesity, diabetes, asthma, abnormal blood profiles, and a history of stroke or seizure.

Proper exercise rarely places us at risk, but you should always take caution. To further help prevent problems for yourself, begin slowly. Use moderate intensity until you feel confident in pushing harder. As I've seen with all of the individuals who have incorporated this program, I'm confident that you'll not only get results, but that you'll also find it to be an enjoyable experience—one that's easy to continue *as a lifestyle.*

Frequently Asked Questions

Q: The *Reclaim 24* weight resistance routine requires me to perform only four high-intensity sets per body part. This is quite different from the old school of thought that suggests many more sets. What's the difference?

A: Most training literature suggests three exercises per body part times three sets per exercise for a total of nine sets. Many athletes perform even a greater number, thinking more must be better. There is no logical or scientific reason for performing so many sets.

Reason and science began to play a role when thinkers such as Arthur Jones, inventor of Nautilus equipment, and Mike Mentzer, champion professional body builder, came on the scene and questioned the validity of such myths. Those two pioneers saw no concrete evidence that performing multiple sets would result in more lean tissue. On the contrary, what they saw was that the overtraining created by executing too many sets often hindered improvement by hurting the body's ability to recuperate. It's during recuperation—rest—that the body repairs and grows muscle (it's called hypertrophy).

With that in mind, it seemed logical to reduce the number of sets to a bare minimum, while performing the sets at a high level of intensity. After all, it's high intensity that stimulates the growth of muscle and lean tissue. When performing too many sets, the exerciser tires before reaching the best level of intensity, minimizing his or her ability to stress a muscle properly for stimulating growth. In other words, the multiple-set theory results in many burned calories but not in the best muscle development.

Whether you want to add muscle size and bulk or simply develop an attractive and toned physique, you require the stimulation of muscle at a high level.

Q: I am a 33 year-old mother of two who is 20 pounds heavier than I was before having children. I am excited about getting back in shape, but I don't wish to look masculine by adding a lot of muscle. Will training with weights make me bulky?

A: Absolutely not! Let's put that age-old myth to rest. Amongst those who have trained with weights for many years, it's quite apparent that adding muscle is no easy task, especially if you're a woman. Weight resistance exercise is the only way to increase muscle and muscle tone, and ultimately change your physique. *Developing size comes from increasing your caloric intake.* If you're restricting calories in an effort to lose fat or control your weight, there is no way you're going to "bulk-up." It's simply not possible to grow larger muscles without adding calories. That's the science. By the way, those women with the perfectly toned bodies seen on the covers of many health magazines look that way because they train with weights.

Q: I've never really been fond of weight training, but I know I must exercise because I am soft and out of shape. Can I develop a nice body taking aerobic classes?

A: Unfortunately not. Please understand that by performing only aerobic exercises, you may improve your cardiovascular health and possibly even keep your overall weight in check. You won't, however, develop shapely, toned muscles to any great extent.

To prove this for yourself, just look at the people in the gym who spend countless hours each week on the treadmill or stationary bike, but who don't train with resistance. Do they ever change? Do they really have the toned, athletic bodies of weight lifters? I don't think so.

Don't be fooled by the TV infomercials showing guys and gals performing exercises on ridiculous exercise equipment that is serving as the fad-of-the-day. That fad equipment did not give them the hard bodies that they display through their skimpy clothing. In truth, they are athletes who train exceptionally hard to develop their physiques. They never, ever use the worthless junk being promoted in the ads.

Q: I've always been told that aerobic exercise burns the most fat. If this is true, then why does the *Reclaim 24* Workout not include this?

A: First of all, aerobic training does indeed have an impact on fat metabolism *while we perform the work*. However, when the work stops, so does most of the extra fat burning! In contrast, muscles are like 24-hour fat-burning engines. Extra muscle growth means an increase in your metabolic rate because muscle, unlike fat, needs calories just for maintenance. This means that added muscle burns calories throughout the day and night, even when the work stops. When you have your cortisol and leptin under control, much of that calorie burning comes from fat.

Although the *Reclaim 24* Workout doesn't seem to incorporate aerobics, it actually does. During the first 30 minutes of the workout, you are performing high-intensity, weight-resistance exercises. To complete the program in 30 minutes, you must move at a rapid pace. This elevates your heart rate throughout the entire 30 minutes to a level achieved with aerobic exercise. So, although you are training with weights, *you receive the benefits of 30 minutes of aerobic training at the same time*. Then, when you add the additional 10 minutes of interval training for further glycogen burn-off, you will have achieved 40 minutes of aerobics. And this occurs three times each week. That is sufficient to keep you aerobically healthy. Of course, if you do any other aerobic activities for fun, that just adds to the numbers.

Q: I've always been told to perform my aerobic exercises to warm up before lifting weights. I noticed that your interval training, which partially replaces low-intensity aerobics, *follows* the weight lifting. Can you explain this?

A: The purpose of interval training is twofold. First, interval training improves cardiovascular fitness and endurance with great efficiency. Second, it's included at the end of the workout to burn off some of the glycogen stores (a form of sugar stored within muscles and the liver) not used by the workout. By initially using glycogen to fuel your weight resistance exercises, you allow for the maximum energy bursts and strength required to grow muscle. Following this, interval training has a tendency to burn through a large portion of the remaining stores. With glycogen largely depleted (but not overly depleted), the body starts using another source of energy *after* your workout ... FAT! You continue to burn a larger percentage of fat until you ingest calories after your workout is finished and a hunger signal arrives. This beats running on the treadmill for 40 minutes straight, don't you think?

Q: My work schedule does not allow me the free time to exercise. What are people in my situation supposed to do?

A: Finding 40 minutes, three times per week is a *choice*. So please be truthful with yourself. If you try hard enough to find excuses, you will. Humans are extraordinarily creative in avoiding things they don't want to do. Getting in shape and caring for your health is either important to you and those you care about or it is not. Only you can decide this. If you're now a person who doesn't have much discipline for following through and maintaining an exercise schedule, then you'll have to find a *purpose* to change. If you cannot find enough reason or purpose within yourself, then think about your family, your significant other, or other loved ones.

Second, if you'll allow it to happen, you'll soon find that dedicating two hours per week to exercise actually increases your energy levels, thereby increasing your productivity. Increased productivity leads to accomplishing more with less time. Any more excuses?

Q: I'm 42 years old and have never been involved in any kind of structured exercise such as weight training. Is it more difficult to develop this habit at my age?

94

A: You're never too old to adopt positive changes in your life. Ending poor habits while simultaneously developing good ones is a matter of bringing some discipline to your mind. It's not about age.

A habit is a habit, whether a good one or a bad one. Developing good habits such as exercise and a life-affirming diet may take time and discipline, but once formed, these habits only get stronger when you see positive changes taking place. You have to decide which habits bring you happiness and which bring you grief, which will bring success and which will simply rob you of precious time and quality of life. Transforming your body into something you can be proud of ultimately leads to transforming your inner-self as well. Once you master the discipline of changing your body, you gain greater mastery in other departments of your life, too.

Q: I am a frequent traveler, which places me in hotels two weeks out of every month. What do you suggest for people like me or for those in the airline industry?

A: Although hotels often don't have much to offer in terms of a variety of exercise equipment, some do. In either case, you can always make best use of what they have available.

If a hotel facility is missing many of the machines or equipment you're used to, you'll find that what they do have can often be used in a variety of ways to train other muscle groups. You might even have to perform a higher number of repetitions if they are limited to only light dumbbells, for example. As long as you follow the principles of the *Reclaim 24* Workout, it's all right to periodically alter your exercises as well as the number of repetitions. Remember, the idea is to attempt to always perform your high-intensity sets to the point of muscle failure. This ensures that your muscles get a sufficient stimulus to respond.

If you don't mind leaving the comforts of your hotel, it's likely you'll find a gym nearby. Almost every city has a variety of nice health clubs that offer up-to-date weight resistance and cardiovascular equipment.

Finally, there are certain lightweight exercise products you can carry *in your luggage* such as exercise bands (www.exercisebands.com— elastic stretch bands with different resistances) or a TRX Suspension Trainer™ (www.fitnessanywhere.com—adjustable straps that use your body's weight as resistance). I talk more about such possibilities on my **www.drcharleswebb.com** website.

Q: A few guys at my health club have pretty large muscular physiques. They appear to train more frequently and far longer than your program suggests. Why is it that they have seemed to put on quality muscle if their type of program leads to overtraining?

A: Yes, it's true that many athletes, mostly men, perform many more sets per body part than what my program calls for. Those same athletes would probably do well with almost any weight resistance program. You see, a few of us are genetically gifted, but most of us are not. The gifted ones have the ability to respond better as well as recuperate more quickly. Some less-gifted folks manage to respond and recuperate better because they use anabolic steroids.

Yet, whether gifted or a user of enhancement drugs, those same athletes would respond *even better* if they used the *Reclaim 24* high-intensity, minimal-sets principles. In other words, they are probably limiting their progress by excessive training, but they fail to realize this because their current program has proven to offer some continued results. They certainly fear losing what they have gained and therefore find it hard to change, especially when the change means performing fewer exercises! In a worst-case scenario, such athletes would maintain their current shapes while freeing up much gym time to work on other aspects of their lives. If only they understood the research and results that others have achieved.... But they are unlikely to heed the science behind muscle development out of fear and habit. Maybe the gym is the only place they can socialize, so it fulfills more than just a bodybuilding or strength-training need.

Remember, one of the main reasons for physical metamorphosis is to learn how to form good habits and carry that knowledge into other—or all—areas of your life. Do you really think it's productive to stay in the gym or exercise longer than necessary? If 40 minutes of training three times a week is enough, then it's enough! Outside of simply enjoying some form of leisure sport, you need to spend your time on other important life activities such as your career, family, mental health, and spiritual health. These things all take much more time than developing your body—and should.

Q: My wife showed her personal trainer your *Reclaim 24* body-shaping program just to get her opinion. Her trainer felt that results would come faster with additional sets and additional time spent on cardio equipment. Do these trainers really know what is best?

A: I can certainly appreciate your wife's curiosity and need for second opinions. I imagine that in starting a new 12-week program, your wife, like most others, would want to tell friends about her new goal and the program that is going to get her there. Her friends, most of them well intentioned I'm sure, would be giving her second opinions. Each would have his or her own idea how to get the best results.

Her personal trainer may also have her own ideas. I know of some trainers who are well educated and thoroughly understand the fundamentals of my program and use it. I'm also aware of many trainers who simply took a quick certification course and magically became experts in the field.

Here's a general bit of advice to help with such issues. Just take a good look at the person giving you the advice and note a couple of things.

1. Does the trainer look to be in good shape? If the people dispensing advice are doing this for their livelihoods, you should expect them to be in good shape, yes?

2. What do their personal clients look like? If the trainers know what they are doing, then a substantial number of their clients will look quite good.

Q: My husband and I have three young children at home. We would really be more comfortable exercising within the home than away at a gym. Can we put together the proper equipment without spending a ton of money?

A: Like many of my friends, I started weight training with little more than a couple of dumbbells (with interchangeable weights) and a bench. With this I was able to develop a well-toned and proportioned physique. The dumbbells supplied all my upper body movements, while I used my own body weight, in the form of one-legged squats, to develop my thighs.

So, the answer is yes! You don't need fancy equipment or a gym membership to obtain your fitness goals. What you do need is Desire, Discipline, and Dedication. Put these three "Ds" together with my high-intensity, body-shaping program and you get the best results possible.

The minimal amount of equipment should include a stable bench, a mat, and a couple of weight-interchangeable dumbbells. If you don't mind spending a few more dollars, you may prefer to purchase five or six sets of dumbbells so you can move more quickly from one set to another.

Q: I've exercised off and on through most of my adult years, but have achieved less than thrilling results for my efforts. Because of this, I find myself quitting altogether for months at a time. How do I maintain my discipline to continue a regular exercise and diet program when I've failed so many times before?

A: I'm glad you brought this up because this is exactly what happens to the majority of men and women who attempt to get into shape. Did you know that over 53% of women and 44% of men fail to make it past three weeks of a structured exercise and diet program? Why such a high failure rate?

Most of us fail, even when loaded with conviction, because the information presently available concerning proper exercise and diet is flat out wrong! It's nothing but a "crapshoot" for most of us when trying to decipher all the conflicting information. Further, food manufacturers willingly take advantage of the current confusion. They exploit loopholes in the food labeling laws to market their junk and make false or misleading claims about their products.

Consider 2% milk, for instance. It's only 2% fat, right? Sounds innocuous enough. But does that mean only 2% of the calories come from fat? Not a chance. If the product is following federal standards for 2% milk, the actual percentage of calories from fat could be 35%.[12] Now that's hardly a low-fat food, is it? Take all of the water out of a gallon of milk and what you have left is a mixture that is 35% fat calories. All of a sudden 2% milk doesn't look like a low-fat food product, does it?

The approach of measuring fat percentage by volume rather than by caloric proportion is what I would call "watering down the public's perceptions." There are countless misleading numbers where that comes from.

With inaccurate and falsified information, how can anyone expect satisfactory results? With the *Reclaim 24* lifestyle program, you develop an enthusiasm to continue improving your physique beyond what you ever anticipated, simply because the program gives you the right information plus a system for *using* the information—and it works!

---

[12] http://www.dairycouncilofca.org/MD_NutritionMain.aspx

10: Rejuvenate with Nourishment

Consuming food is, and always will be, pleasurable for healthy people. You deserve enjoyment. But not at the expense of your health! I'll have to admit that dining out is common in my lifestyle and has been for years. It's tough to beat a night out socializing with friends and being served a fabulous meal that would have taken more time to prepare than to consume. And that doesn't even count cleanup time.

For as far back as history reveals, social events have been associated with meals. Today, eating still serves as a social medium for all cultures and personalities as a part of celebrations, business lunches, and everything in-between. Mealtime seems to magically bring people together in a more peaceful setting, no matter what their differences might be.

Should You Eat for Pleasure?

Eating definitely has a soothing effect on us that temporarily allows us to forget our troubles. This isn't a bad thing if we don't get into the habit of attacking the refrigerator every time we have a tough day. Too many people do that often enough to create problems for themselves.

Do you recall in Chapter 4 when I talked about the reasons human beings make the choices they do? We're trying to either gain pleasure or avoid pain. So when you eat, are you eating because you're truly hungry or are you simply looking for some pleasure?

Don't panic; neither answer is wrong! It's okay to eat for pleasure as long as that temporary pleasure doesn't contribute to pain later on. You know what I mean. If you have to scarf down a slice of double chocolate cake after a filling meal just for pleasure, you'll probably begin to feel a tinge of guilt (emotional pain) not long after. Now, the only reason you feel the guilt is that you realize where that chocolate cake will ultimately end up. The emotional pain lasts a lot longer than consumption of the cake!

I enjoy a slice of chocolate cake every occasionally. There's room for that in my eating lifestyle once one's metabolism can handle it. The key is to enjoy it infrequently. You'll be happy to know that my nutritional approach allows for a "cheat day," every four or five days, so there's no need to stress out just yet.

Again, eating is pleasurable and should be. But can't it also be a pleasurable experience for you while eating the right kinds of foods? Are you able to enjoy ingesting the foods that actually have life-creating value instead of those with empty calories and no vitality? Of course you are able. It's a matter of changing habits—perhaps habits that you've held to for many years.

This might be a good time to re-read the beginning of Chapter 5, "Breaking Old Habits." You might easily be saying to yourself right about now, "Eating healthy is boring, and I simply don't have the time to prepare all my meals that way." Well first, eating healthy is quite pleasurable—or becomes pleasurable—because you can enjoy the true flavors of natural foods without the added fat, sugar, or both. Second, preparing healthful dishes takes less time than preparing the meals that grandma did. I know grandma cooked great meals, but if you consider the butter in the potatoes and lard in the pies, they weren't healthful. Besides, look at the mess you had to clean up.

Believe me, cooking healthy is the way to go if you are the family's elected dishwasher. And for those of you who also enjoy eating out, whether fine dining or a quick lunch, you'll be glad to know healthful choices are available to you. Both fine-dining and fast-food establishments now commonly offer healthful alternatives. When these alternatives are not offered, the waiter can usually alter the item of your choice to reduce calories and fat. Ask for salad dressing on the side and avoid dishes made with cheese or heavy sauces.

Support for the Continuous Creation of Life

We eat for many reasons, but few of us give much thought to the actual life-creating processes that are supported by the nutrients we ingest. Selecting the right foods is a choice you have to make more frequently if you're planning for success in your body and health metamorphosis. Today, we also know that *when* you eat those right foods is more important than ever.

If you are to begin changing your eating habits, you need a general understanding of the importance of nutrients. Proper nutrients offer the environment for healthy cell regeneration. You can't feel it, but your body is constantly replacing old, worn-out cells with new ones. Every year your body replaces about 90% of its cells, creating an almost totally new you! Doesn't it make sense that cell replacement should occur under the best of conditions?

Empty calorie foods such as refined, processed products don't offer any real value to the biological chain of events that brings yearly physical renewal. Only vital, life-creating nutrients found in whole foods can fuel this continued rebirth of the body. When new cells receive the proper ingredients to remain healthy, the aging process is slowed. In contrast, the intake of poor, denatured foods accelerates the aging process quite a bit, especially after age 30. If this isn't reason enough to clean up your diet, I don't know what is.

Look at it this way. Day after day, you have the ability to make choices that can help maintain the glow of your youth. This includes vitality, energy, sex drive, appealing body composition, and a clear mind. To think you can have all this simply by choosing the right foods over the wrong ones should make your decision easy. And it becomes easier for you with time and some substitutions in habit.

Fuel for Energy and Growth

The Reclaim 24 program involves eating the right foods at the right times, getting ample nutrients and calories to support the lean tissue growth you need, deriving efficient *energy* from your food, and watching your level of wellness rise with each passing month. And how do we do that?

Well, if you read the first edition of this book entitled *Reclaim 24*, you know I advocated eating five or six small meals a day to provide continuous nutrition for boosting metabolism, to assure that nutrients are consistently available, and to avoid blood sugar imbalances. That six-meals-per-day approach has been the common nutritional wisdom among a certain cadre of thinkers for at least several decades now. But like any common wisdom, it can be turned on its head with new scientific discoveries. After all, at one time the common wisdom for treating scurvy was to burn the afflicted at the stake. And bloodletting was popular for nearly 2000 years.

"Many children, teenagers, young adults, intense bodybuilders, and athletes can seemingly [eat six small meals per day] without any apparent consequence. This is because their demand for calories to aid body growth and repair is quite high. This genetic gift tends to disappear after age thirty. However, it is alarming the number of children who are

overweight and too inactive, and who thus have hormonal balance problems that used to be present only in the over-thirty age group." [13]

I'm now convinced the wisdom of eating five or six small meals a day has been turned on its head for all except complicated diabetics, hypoglycemics, and the exceptions just mentioned. We are now back to three squares a day, five to six hours apart, *with no snacking in between*. Here's why.

Since the time I published my first edition explaining Reclaim 24, intensive research into the recently discovered (1994) hormone, **leptin**, has been more rapidly making its way into the nutritional mainstream, as detailed by Byron Richards.[14] Indeed, nutritional and metabolic science has been looking at the extremely complex interplay between adrenaline, insulin, and leptin. It's now clear that the timing and composition of meals is crucial if we are to retain balance among these hormones and prevent insulin, leptin, and adrenaline resistance in our tissues—with special emphasis on leptin resistance. Such resistances mean we are losing control of our health and wellness, and we need to get to the bottom of it.

As Richards explains, we are starting to see that there is *one* healthy way to eat for nearly all of us. *"It is a way that maximizes the efficient function of leptin. All this information is new. Low-fat diets are incredibly destructive, as are high-fat diets. Understanding leptin finally puts to rest the conflicting diet information that is currently running rampant in society."* [15] Furthermore, he says, *"The food pyramid, even though its creators may have been well intentioned, is an eating method that induces serious health issues."* Indeed, the Government Food Pyramid places way too much emphasis on eating carbohydrates relative to protein. The very recent replacement for the Food Pyramid, the Food Plate, does somewhat better.

Twenty-first century discoveries about leptin and its role in our metabolism have dramatically changed thinking about meal frequency and wellness practice. If you're having a battle with unwanted fat deposits and energy depletion, you will have to develop a few good habits to get your body's energy metabolism back on track. Anyone who wishes to retain wellness as the calendar years add up will need to understand how to do this.

---

[13] Richards, Byron J., with Mary Guignon Richards, *Mastering Leptin: Your Guide to Permanent Weight Loss and Permanent Health,* Third Edition, Wellness Resources Books, p. 138.

[14] Ibid. A groundbreaking book, not easy to assimilate in one reading, but groundbreaking nonetheless.

[15] Ibid, p. 5

Why? According to Richards' extensive research, it's because, chronic problems with leptin balance set the stage for serious health issues down the road. In addition to obesity, these health issues include heart disease, cancer, anorexia, and bone loss. As well, they include immune, gastrointestinal, liver, nerve, and cognitive problems. That's sure a lot of problems.

Rules and Strategies for Leptin Management

This book is not the best place to cite *too* many details about leptin chemistry and metabolism, although I will say a little more about it in chapter 14. If you have the incentive to dig deeper, you can get further details by contacting your wellness professional, by reading Richards' book on leptin, or both,. For now, I'd just like to point you in the right direction concerning leptin management.

The best place to start is with Richards' five dietary rules for managing leptin. These rules apply to almost everyone, perhaps with exception of some diabetics or the intense calorie users mentioned earlier. Teaching yourself (and your metabolism) to follow these rules consistently should be an integral part of your wellness practice because they help you avoid upsetting your energy metabolism and losing your health. The rules reflect habits that serve for a lifetime, no matter what your age. Of course, the earlier you start, the better. You'll be able to reverse stress damage more quickly. So here they are, straight from Richards' book: [16]

Rule 1: **Never eat after dinner. Allow eleven to twelve hours between dinner and breakfast. Never go to bed on a full stomach. Finish eating dinner at least three hours before bed.**

Rule 2: **Eat three meals a day. Allow five to six hours between meals. Do not snack. (See exceptions starting p. 101).**

Rule 3: **Do not eat large meals. If you are overweight, always try to finish a meal when you are slightly less than full; the full signal will usually catch up in ten to twenty minutes. Eating slowly is important.**

Rule 4: **Eat a breakfast containing protein.**

Rule 5: **Reduce the amount of carbohydrates you eat.**

---

[16] Ibid, p. 115.

You may read those rules, especially the first and second, and say to yourself, "Yikes! I can't do that. My body doesn't work that way." But guess what. That's your out-of-balance leptin metabolism putting words in your mouth! It's saying, "I'm in control now, not you!" If you accept that metabolic decree as your life sentence, you are riding the Conveyor Belt to a Living Hell. If you don't accept it, however, you can slowly shift your metabolism towards greater health by managing your diet and eating patterns, taking the right supplements, managing your stress and hormone levels, exercising properly, and engaging in appropriate forms of detoxification (see chapter 16).

Here's an important excerpt from Richards' book:[17]

> Some individuals may need to gradually work their eating in the right direction. They may need to have four meals a day, four hours apart. As they increase their exercise and improve the condition of the pancreas, adrenals, muscles, and liver, they will gradually be able to move to the three-meal-a-day plan without their energy dropping between meals.
>
> If five to six small meals a day are needed to maintain energy, the metabolic situation is not in good shape. Eating very small meals may cause some weight loss, but metabolism will likely slow down before the weight goal is achieved. Even a low-calorie snack increases insulin release; thus fat-burning mode ceases or never begins. Only by increasing the amount of time between meals will proper weight loss take place.

Please remember one thing that Richards points out: If you cannot follow a rule, it doesn't mean the rule is wrong! There are creative ways for you to ease your way towards your goal of being able to follow the five rules. You didn't get into your state of leptin and insulin resistance overnight, so it may take you a while to reverse it. If it's too difficult to go it alone, you'll do best with the help of a qualified wellness professional who knows about leptin metabolism.

* * *

So, other than stubborn weight around the middle, what does it look like when your leptin metabolism is unbalanced? You might be surprised. Here's a shortlist of signs and symptoms:

---

[17] Ibid, pp. 137–138

Common Signs & Symptoms that Your
Leptin Metabolism is Out of Control

- You are 15 or more pounds above your ideal weight.

- You have an out-of-control appetite after dinner, perhaps right up until bedtime. You simply overeat. This is the single, most important symptom telling you your leptin metabolism is out of control.

- If you don't eat before bed, you can't get to sleep; or you wake up with a headache or feel queasy. Or, if you don't have a nighttime snack, you wake up hungry in the middle of the night.

- You are unable to eat breakfast or are not hungry in the morning for up to two or three hours.

- You do eat in the morning, but it's typically something like a sweet roll, muffin, or orange juice—probably with coffee, too.

- You regularly desire something sweet or something fat that overwhelms your willpower (hormone imbalances are larger than willpower).

- You do not feel satisfied eating a normal amount of food. You may feel quite irritable and think you won't have any energy until you eat more.

- It's impossible for you to go five hours without eating between meals, e.g., breakfast to lunch. You need to snack between meals.

- You eat too many carbohydrates, such as cookies for lunch.

- Your head is not clear or you lack vibrant energy.

- Your (digital) weight scale reads higher at night than in the morning.

- You've lost the desire to do something about being overweight because you've failed so many times in the past.

- You can become irrational about getting food until you get the "fix" that you need. Then you can think rationally one again.

- You're not getting regular exercise.

Do you recognize anything in that list?

* * *

Although nature often *seems* to overlook the negative lifestyle habits of "teenies" and "20 somethings," that illusion evaporates ever so quickly as we move into our 30's and beyond. By the time we reach 40, rules and strategies for leptin management become mandatory. Coasting is no longer an option. If you don't pay serious, conscious attention to what you are doing, the stress buildup, systemic inflammation, and energy depletion that comes from leptin, insulin, and adrenaline resistance takes over and your journey along the Conveyor Belt to a Living Hell becomes a foregone conclusion.

On the other hand, if you learn to manage leptin with awareness and intelligence, you can forestall or prevent such stress buildup well into your senior years. It's your choice. But calendar age is *not* a legitimate excuse for allowing stress to build up more quickly once you leave your 20's. You now know better, or you shall by the time you finish reading this book.

So what have we been learning lately in leptin science? Especially about our attempts at weight loss? Or about maintaining our fat composition at a healthy, desirable level? Well, for one thing, the primitive side of your brain has its own "ideas" about how much fat you should carry, and those ideas are not negotiable. They express themselves in drives and overpowering urges in which leptin plays a part.

The fact is your primitive brain—the subconscious part—does not consult your conscious mind about what you want to see when you look into a full-length mirror. Nor does it even know, for sure, how much fat you already have on board! It can only rely on signals from the fat, itself, being delivered properly. Those are leptin signals, if you must know. If leptin signals don't get through to the brain as well as they should because of resistance, the brain automatically orders the liver to store more fat with the help of the pancreas and insulin.

So what factor is actually at play within your primitive brain? It is *your survival instinct,* or at least your survival as your subconscious, primitive brain perceives or measures it. Your subconscious is genetically in charge of your survival at a molecular level, and if it "concludes" that your life is at stake because of perceived starvation, it will send out commands to eat more. It will create, store, and hold onto fat with a tenacity that defies all your efforts at turning things around. In the meantime, it will slow your metabolism, energy levels, and immune response to a crawl so that the fat you have stored will hang around as long as possible.

Unbelievably, just the *thought* of dieting by those who have already suffered through one or more unsuccessful diets in the past is sufficient to trigger the subconscious to kick into more eating and fat conservation. To the energy metabolism center of the brain, to diet is to starve. The more yo-yo dieting you've done in the past, the quicker and easier it is for the brain's primitive protection mechanism to kick into action. Unless you learn how to balance your leptin metabolism as part of your lifestyle, you simply will not be able to reach *and maintain* your goal weight—the weight that means a lifetime of wellness for you.

And one more thing. Your subconscious pays little if any attention to your conscious willpower to diet; or to your desire to restrict yourself from eating or craving certain foods. You probably already know this from having experienced terrific urges to eat something sweet or something with fat. Once an urge turns on, there's no turning it off. Try to fight it and the urge will even follow you into your dreams, where you'll find yourself eating the things you crave! Finally, you just give in.

In truth, it's frightfully easy for the primitive subconscious to overcome the force of your willpower. You cannot win this battle of leptin "misbehavior" with willpower, alone, unless you are already close to having a state of balance. Then you can readily adopt the five rules. Otherwise, the only way you can win is to prevent it from happening in the first place. This will require knowledge, imagination, a plan for reversing long-term damage, and proper action. You already learned something about how and why the subconscious rules your behavior in chapter 6: "How the Subconscious Mind Works to Help or Hurt You." Those subconscious principles also apply to your attempts to diet or control eating urges.

Here's the point. Hormonal signals that control energy metabolism pass between your brain, fat tissue, muscle tissue, liver, pancreas, and adrenals. If those signals get out of whack, you will no longer have control over what you look like (size-wise), how much energy you have, how clearly you think, how well your immune system works, or how quickly the Conveyor Belt to a Living Hell carries you to its destination. Your willpower will have darn little to say about it unless you begin to intelligently direct that willpower towards changing the habits that are slowly destroying your quality of life (and maybe even killing you).

Scientifically, it's beginning to look like leptin signals are the mother of all signals! So that's where you must look, first, if you are having trouble with urges and too much fat storage.

* * *

If you correctly exercise and stimulate lean tissue growth, your body needs ample nutrients and calories to support that growth. Skipping meals not only hinders this growth process but also creates a "starvation response" that leads to a slower metabolism. And it all starts with breakfast.

Never, ever miss breakfast, *even if you're not hungry!* Metabolically, it is the most important meal of the day. Studies show that people who eat breakfast feel better both mentally and physically than those who skip their morning meal. They feel perkier. British researchers at Cardiff University even found that eating breakfast is associated with lower levels of the stress hormone cortisol.

> Never, ever miss breakfast, *even if you're not hungry!* This is the most important meal of the day. It 'kick-starts' your metabolism and helps protect you from hormonal imbalances.

People who say they "can't eat breakfast" usually get that way because their leptin signaling has gone awry and they habitually eat late at night. Now I'm not suggesting that you "force feed" yourself, but you can always eat a small portion of something nutritious in the morning, especially something with protein content. You'll discover that it really pays dividends in how you feel. You'll also find it easier to control your weight and to follow the five rules for maintaining leptin balance, especially the rule against eating after dinner.

Indeed, breakfast "kick-starts" your metabolism. However, it shouldn't include typical breakfast foods such as cereal, pastries, and juice. These foods only send your blood sugar through the roof, forcing your pancreas into overdrive. They also mess up your leptin metabolism for the day so that your satiation signals don't work after dinner. Over time, this can lead to insulin resistance, leptin resistance, adrenaline resistance, and adult-onset diabetes. Instead, choose protein-rich foods such as eggs, lean meats, or even a protein supplement along with complex carbohydrates found in oatmeal or oat bran. Try to add some high fiber, *whole* fruit such as apples or pears. These types of foods do not cause your blood sugar to rise too rapidly unless you are quite unhealthy. Moreover, these foods are more efficient for growing lean tissue rather than fat tissue.

Did you know that as you age, lean tissue mass is better maintained by foods rich in potassium—fruits and vegetables?[18] Yet, many older folks move towards a greater intake of sugars and grains, exactly the opposite of what is best for them. Take heed if you want to practice wellness! And if you really want to break some molds, start thinking about eating high-fiber vegetables at breakfast instead of large quantities of sugars, starches, and grains. American dietary habits are really quite silly when you think about it.

Quality versus Quantity

As Americans, we have had the blessing of plentiful food. This has also turned out to be somewhat of a curse. We don't have to spend any time hunting, gathering or even preparing if we choose not to. All we have to do is drive through the fast-food lane and answer the question, "Do you want fries with that?" Presto! You have a fully prepared hot meal that includes 10% of your daily protein, 100% of your daily fat, 60% of your daily carbohydrates, and all in just 1,200 calories.

Sounds crazy, doesn't it? Well, that's an all-too-typical scenario for nearly 70% of us living in this country. Americans are obese because these highly processed, high-caloric foods have become diet staples. Granted, most of us also fail because we don't participate in any kind of vigorous activity or exercise program. However, I can say with complete confidence that even exercise can't counter the effects of these high-calorie, low-nutrition diets. They are slow poisons to our systems. They promote slow suicide.

Sitting down to eat a Big Mac®, fries, and a Coke won't necessarily fill you up any more than a turkey sandwich and a salad. Both meals require about the same time to consume, and both stretch our stomachs about the same. So why is it that the person eating the turkey sandwich probably fulfills his or her hunger needs while the person eating the Big Mac more than likely won't? Although the McDonald's meal contains roughly twice the calories, the calories are predominately processed carbohydrates and saturated fats.

Processed carbohydrates quickly enter the bloodstream causing insulin spikes. Because these kinds of carbohydrates are absorbed and assimilated so easily, the body does not need to use any of the fat for

---

[18] Dawson-Hughes B., Harris S.S., Ceglia L., "Alkaline Diets Favor Lean Tissue Mass in Older Adults," Am J Clin Nutr. 2008 Mar;87(3):662-5.

immediate energy. So the extra calories get stored as more fat. With repeated and prolonged insulin spikes, our cells start to become resistant to insulin. This means the body needs more insulin to do the same job it was doing before with less. In a sense, body cells become insulin "addicts" and require more and more to be satisfied. This leads to adult-onset diabetes. Further, with prolonged, elevated levels of insulin, an associated metabolic shift in cortisol levels occurs. This shift also leads to leptin resistance through other metabolic processes. And since leptin is responsible for appetite suppression, resistance to its effects will mean hunger doesn't get satisfied even though plenty of calories have been consumed.

To summarize this in nonprofessional terms, fast food is generally higher in calories, stores itself as fat more readily, and does not suppress your appetite as well as nutrient-rich, unprocessed food. But Americans can't get enough of the fast stuff! This is why the option to "SUPER SIZE" became so popular. Who ever heard of "SUPER SIZING" a deli-sandwich-and-soup meal?

So, as you may have gathered, I'm not asking you to eat less food, just less calorie-laden, heavily processed food. Wouldn't it be more rewarding to eat three meals of 500 calories each than one fast-food meal of 1,500 calories? Your hormone balance will love it, as will your physique or figure.

Do you think you can't find low-calorie, nutrient-rich food within the fast-food chains? I regularly eat lunch away from home and find no problem in staying away from hamburgers, fries, and tacos. As things currently stand, Subway offers whole wheat breads, a variety of lean meats, and close to a dozen choices of vegetables. Chick fil-A® offers a grilled chicken breast on a whole-wheat bun, served with a bowl of fruit and bottled water. Most chain restaurants have "heart smart" meals that usually consist of lean meats and vegetables while minimizing processed pastas and white bread. There simply is no excuse to blame lack of availability for your choices.

Okay, we've covered the advantages of nutrient-rich foods. Now is a good time to delve into more detail about nutrients.

P.S. Chapter 10: Did you know that if you have a cup of coffee in the morning before eating breakfast, the cortisol spike may keep you from burning fat for the rest of the day?

11: The Nutrients and Other Dietary Essentials

I'll preface this chapter by saying that research in health and nutrition, along with the eye-opening reevaluation of old research, has been moving at a blistering pace. Any information that you can find in a new book is likely to be obsolescent even before the book reaches your hands. That's how things are these days. *Fast.*

But somehow we must find ways to keep pace if we're interested in wellness, remembering that those not interested in wellness are at an extraordinary disadvantage in maintaining health and staying of the Conveyor Belt to a Living Hell. I wish I could say that everything in this book is right on the money in terms of its currency and efficacy, but I can't. I've done my absolute best to make it so in both editions, but I'm also a realist who knows that health information grows beyond us ever so quickly. Such has been the case with our knowledge of leptin.

As another example, recent findings indicate that the sweetener, sucralose (Splenda®) may not be the innocuous, wonderful product that it's promoted to be. Further, too much tuna in the diet may not be a good idea because of mercury contamination. How can we possibly keep up with such information in reasonable ways?

How to Keep up with the Latest Health Information

As bad a reputation as the Internet has gotten (and deserved) in some cases, *it's also the most likely place to find the best, most current information on health and nutrition.* So I'm going to recommend just two websites for you to follow *at the outset* to help you avoid riding off on your horse in a dozen directions or feeling that the top of your head might pop off from information overload and conflicting viewpoints. Of course, these websites are certainly not the only sources of information on wellness, but they are wonderful places to start. You'll be able to retain your sanity as you gain a foothold. With time, you'll find yourself in a better position to spread your wings as you learn more about wellness practice and follow your educated hunches about what might be right for you and what might not. These websites are:

> www.drcharleswebb.com—This is my website for *Reclaim 24* support. It complements this book. I make every effort to keep the site current and tremendously helpful for those

looking to enhance wellness in their lives by understanding and actually practicing it! I work diligently to keep current with the latest and greatest information and discoveries.

www.mercola.com—This is one of the Web's most visited and trusted health and wellness information sites. It's run by Dr. John Mercola, a doctor of osteopathy (DO) who has full medical training. However, in the early years of his practice he concluded that wellness practice offers more health than the practice of conventional medicine. He has a passion not only for myth busting but also for breaking the existing medical and drug establishment's perilous and self-serving holds in this country. His site is always at the *leading edge of health discoveries* and other interesting revelations, as is his free e-newsletter. Sure, he has his own slant toward helping the health-seeking public get out from under the thumb of wellness ignorance, but so what? Everybody has a slant, even those who claim immaculate objectivity. The information on the Mercola site is there for our benefit if we want to practice wellness. And though controversial in some circles, it's proven time and again to be generally good information.

www.WellnessResources.com/leptin—An excellent place to do your leptin research. The website is run by the author of *Mastering Leptin,* Byron Richards.

Well that's it for my best, most practical recommendations for keeping up as you dip your toe into the waters of optimized living. You don't want to throw such opportunities away because wellness practice is a full-time, full-contact sport!

Carbohydrates (4 calories per gram)

In the past few years, carbohydrates have been labeled the primary culprit in America's obesity epidemic. Here is the thought process: eliminate carbs and you eliminate obesity. To further push this epidemic into a tailspin, the public is being taught that it's okay to load up on a high protein, high fat diet as long as we cut out potatoes and bread. So, people are now replacing their bread with high-caloric foods such as cheese and bacon, thinking this makes sense. I'm sorry, but this is madness, and the cost is high.

It's true that ingesting certain types of carbohydrates is one of the main reasons for obesity in this country, but drastically eliminating carbohydrates does not solve the problem. Fruits and high-fiber vegetables are carbohydrates. Does it make sense to replace these nutrient- and antioxidant-rich foods with high-caloric dairy products or pig fat? If it weren't for fruits and vegetables, we would suffer many health problems from lack of nutrients and fiber. And we'd "age" much more quickly.

Ingesting more fiber-rich fruits and vegetables only has a positive effect on your health, while simultaneously helping you shed unwanted body fat. Go ahead—try to get fat while taking most of your calories in the form of whole fruits and vegetables. It's difficult. These foods are typically low in calories while high in fiber and water. This means it's tough to consume too many calories before getting full. Even with most fruit, which has a higher concentration of natural sugar (calories) than vegetables, we tend to fill up easily and don't have the ongoing cravings associated with processed carbohydrates.

However, major problems have arisen through assumptions about fructose, the dominant sugar in fruit and some vegetables. What can possibly be bad about fruit sugar, right? It's so natural! It was also thought to be healthy when introduced in large quantities as a sweetener.

Although classified as a simple sugar, fructose does not require the same demands on the pancreas hormone, insulin, as do other sugars—especially processed sugars. In other words, it creates less insulin spiking from a meal because it a "low glycemic index" food. That's the upside. But everything goes downhill from there, and fast—especially if you don't get your fructose from whole fruits and vegetables.

Processed fructose—abundantly present in high-fructose corn syrup (HFCS) in order to make it sweeter—has *many* more metabolic negatives than other types of sugar, including its penchant to raise cholesterol and serum triglyceride levels. As you know, elevated levels of these substances are high-risk factors for heart disease. Worse still, because fructose is not metabolized in the same way as other sugars (it converts to ethanol), it doesn't trigger the appetite-suppression mechanism. It leaves those who consume it feeling unsatisfied so they keep eating.

Growing evidence says that fructose in abundance promotes insulin resistance by back-door means, eventually leading to type-2 diabetes. Moreover, *HFCS converts to fat in the body more easily than any other*

113

type of sugar. Large quantities of fructose (74+ grams)—just 2 ½ sugary soft drinks a day[19]—cause the liver to pump fats into the bloodstream that may damage arteries. Such quantities also raise the risk of high blood pressure.

HFCS is downright ornery because it is present in so many places in the American food supply. It's dirt-cheap to manufacture. In addition to being used as a sugar substitute, we find it in many processed foods and beverages, including soft drinks, yogurt, industrial bread, cookies, salad dressings, and even tomato soup. It's everywhere! And people's livers are being overwhelmed by it. When this happens, livers immediately turn it into triglicerides and release it into the blood to be stored as fat. HFCS *is now believed to be the primary culprit for the obesity epidemic that we see around us.* The observed correlation between the growing use of HFCS and the obesity/diabetes epidemic is compelling.

By the way, the recent upstart, agavé syrup, also called agavé nectar, is even higher in processed fructose than HFCS. Agavé is marketed as a natural, healthy, low-glycemic-index sweetener. Well, it's not natural or healthy, no matter what the marketers say. It is a highly processed fructose product, sometimes even "watered down" with HFCS to make it cheaper to manufacture. Again, *it is not natural!* It goes through much processing to deliver its high level of sweetness.

Having said that, unless you're diabetic or have developed insulin resistance (which many people don't recognize), *you don't need to monitor your intake of fructose so long as you are getting it from eating whole fruits and vegetables.* Fructose ingested as part of its whole food component is mostly innocuous. Fruit juice, on the other hand, is extremely high in calories. You should always monitor its intake. Fructose-intense drinks—including many sodas—are slow, steadfast killers. As far as the processed- and fast-food industries are concerned, the slower they kill you, the better. More sales before you go.

By the way, have you seen recent ads on TV promoting the "naturalness" of HFCS because it's starting to take the heat? That's your processed food industry at work, trying to keep you hooked on a bad, bad food additive. Don't fall for it. They aren't telling the whole story.

* * *

---

[19] News release, American Society of Nephrology, Oct. 29, 2009

Overall, we need complex carbohydrates in our diet. We can break these into three categories:

Starch—Potatoes, grains, and legumes
Fiber—Wheat bran, oat bran, and vegetable cellulose
Glycogen—Quick-release, high-energy fuel stored natively in muscles and the liver

As you can see, this list includes some of the foods we have recently been taught are bad for us, i.e. potatoes and bread. Yes, bread is a processed food; however, non-fortified, whole-grain products offer essential nutrients and fiber when not sweetened with HFCS. Neither potatoes nor HFCS-free whole-grain breads are bad for people who have retained good insulin and leptin sensitivity, especially if the breads are gluten free. They just don't belong with every meal. And when it comes to potatoes, try to enjoy them without frying or putting all the junk on them. A typical potato has only about 150 calories.

By far, your best source of complex carbohydrates comes from fibrous vegetables.[20] You should be getting plenty of them in your diet.

Carbohydrates serve as the body's main fuel source. Proteins and fats must be converted to glucose within the liver before the body can burn them, while complex carbohydrates are easily broken down to simple sugars that the body can use immediately.

The types of carbohydrates responsible for America's bulge are mainly the processed variety. What are processed carbohydrates? Just about any food that comes in a box, a wrapper, or in the form of bottled drinks other than water. This may be too simplistic in some regards, but certainly paints a reasonable picture for a shopper interested in moving towards wellness practice. Stay away from anything in a box, wrapper, or drink bottle and you're already way out in front. Forego baked goods (cakes, brownies, rolls, biscuits), cereals (Wheaties®, Cap'n Crunch®, raisin bran), white pasta (macaroni and cheese), prepared sweets (cookies, candy bars, cinnamon crackers), sodas, juices, and other sweetened drinks. Just by eliminating the foods in boxes, wrappers, and drink bottles, you eliminate the majority of processed foods.

---

[20] The list is very long, but vegetables highest in fiber include avocado, beans, broccoli, brussels sprouts, lentils, cabbage, carrot, chick peas (garbanzo beans), eggplant, greens (collards, kale, turnip), lima beans, mushrooms, potato with skin, pumpkin (canned), black-eyed peas, green peas, peppers, rhubarb, spinach, and sweet potatoes.

Now, I'm not saying that *all* boxed or wrapped foods or bottled drinks are off limits. Just keep them to a minimum if you want to get results that last. You'll note that processed carbohydrates, unlike fruits and vegetables, can live on a store shelf quite nicely without canning or refrigeration. The fact that insects won't eat them says a lot!

Most processed carbohydrates have minimal nutrient value and are loaded with sugar. As I mentioned earlier, this sugar creates havoc in the body's ability to control blood sugar or glucose levels. Over time, this leads to the loss of insulin and leptin sensitivity, and a diminished ability to use glucose. Although fructose (usually from high-fructose corn syrup) won't raise your glucose levels as much as other sugars in a meal, it has devastating consequences in ways that I mentioned earlier, including raising insulin levels with long-term ingestion. Processed carbohydrates are also high in calories and don't promptly satiate the appetite. It's easy to eat too much before you realize you're full. The result, of course, is fat buildup.

Recommended Daily Intake of Carbohydrates

So, just how much of your daily food consumption should be made up of carbohydrates? About 40–65% of all the calories you consume should be in the form of complex or high-fiber carbohydrates. Where in that range you fall depends on whether you're attempting to lose weight, maintain your weight, or pack on some additional muscle. Caloric intake must flex according to your goal, while the total grams of protein you ingest depend on your body weight. Here's a summary of the recommended carbohydrate percentages.

- Grow muscle
  - 55-65% of total calories
- Maintain weight
  - 50-55% of total calories
- Lose weight (fat)
  - 40-50% of total calories

Carbohydrate Myths

Myth 1: Carbohydrates make you fat.
  Fact: Excessive calories and leptin resistance make you fat.
  Fact: Processed carbohydrates make you fat because they harm your leptin sensitivity.

116

Myth 2: All carbohydrates are alike.

    Fact: Complex carbohydrates slow down digestion a bit, don't spike insulin levels as much, and are usually more nutritious.

    Fact: Processed carbohydrates increase the demand on the pancreas. A continuous demand leads to adult-onset diabetes.

Myth 3: Low carbohydrate foods are preferable.

    Fact: Low carbohydrate foods are often high in fat.

    Fact: High-fiber *vegetables* are low in fat and carbohydrates.

Protein (4 calories per gram)

One can't overstate the importance of protein. If you're to succeed in changing your body composition for the better, which means to lean out and tone up, you *must* eat enough protein. Protein provides the building blocks (amino acids) for tissue building.

The average American diet is lacking in good sources of protein. Sure, most of us are not vegetarians and do consume meat, which is a complete source of protein, but often the grade of meat isn't so good (excess fat and loaded with hormones). Don't kid yourself into thinking that the hamburgers served at fast-food joints are of high or even moderate quality. In truth, I highly recommend that you avoid them entirely.

On the other hand, whole breast of chicken or turkey is pretty much the same no matter who is serving it. Aside from how it's prepared, the fowl itself is lean and offers a complete source of protein. The main recommendation here, as with all animal and fowl products, is to avoid consuming products not fed and raised organically. Why is that? Because most supermarket and restaurant meats are raised with synthetic hormones that can build up within your system when eaten. These hormones, mostly estrogens, tend to block hormone receptor sites within your glands and prevent normal hormonal function. These synthetic hormones are called *endocrine disruptors*. They play a major role in contributing to the obesity epidemic.

What about good old-fashioned red meat? Sure, why not? Red meat is an excellent source of amino acids and contains important vitamins not found in other foods. The only downfall with red meat is that it contains a larger percentage of saturated fat than chicken and most fish. At high intake levels, saturated fat is thought to lead to cardiovascular disease, but that's no longer clear. To stay out of trouble, simply choose the lean variety, and eat it in moderation. Again, choose only organic varieties—and preferably grass-fed—when eating at home.

If you really want to improve your ability to burn fat while getting a superior source of protein, choose fish, especially the variety that is high in omega-3 fatty acids (the good kind of fat). Wild Alaskan salmon is by far the best choice since it has the perfect ratio of omega 3's to omega-6's—1:2. I mention the wild version because, compared with the farmed variety, it if of higher quality and contains less-toxic PCBs and lower levels of saturated fat. Tilapea, on the other hand, is most often farmed and fed foods that not only make it fatty, but also make it too high in omega 6. Best avoided in quantity.

Other good choices of fish include "light" tuna (best kept to about two cans per week because of latent mercury levels), mackerel, sardines, and sablefish. Unfortunately, fish isn't a staple of the American diet. Nor is it ever likely to be. I haven't seen many fast-food chains that offer fish, except perhaps those that specialize in deep frying. I don't really consider patrons of such establishments to be fish lovers.

For those who enjoy fish as a main protein source, please stay informed about mercury levels in particular types of fish. In recent years, poisons have managed to make their way into the flesh of our swimming friends because of contaminants and pollutants being poured into our streams and rivers. Unfortunately, these same poisons can affect us. All I'm saying is to be responsible for your health and try to stay informed if you consume a moderate amount of fish or crustaceans. In any case, do try to include fish in your diet. It's good for you.

You can get your daily quota of protein without depending solely on meat. Primary sources of both complete proteins (all of the essential amino acids are present) and incomplete proteins include:

Animal Proteins – Meat, milk, and eggs (organic preferred)
- o   Contain all the amino necessary acids (complete)
- o   Longer digestion and absorption time

Plant Proteins – legumes and nuts
- o   Incomplete source of amino acids
- o   Slow digestion and absorption time

You may note that soy is missing from plant proteins. And for good reason. Recent research has been showing that soy isn't nearly the health food that's it's promoted to be. For example, soy protein is high in phytoestrogens, which are *endocrine disruptors*. For safety, avoid using unfermented[21] soy products. This isn't so easy because soy has been sneaking its way into many foods as a meat substitute and protein booster. It's so cheap! Soy is often hidden on labels as something else; for example, textured vegetable protein, soy protein isolate, lecithin, or vegetable oil. In truth, soy, in an unfermented state, may be quite harmful to the body over long periods. Thousands of studies link soy to malnutrition, digestive distress, immune-system breakdown, thyroid dysfunction, cognitive decline, reproductive disorders, and infertility— even cancer and heart disease. Hard to believe, yes?

With regard to infant soy formulas, the estrogens in soy can irreversibly harm a baby's future sexual development and reproductive health. The negatives go on and on, but commercial interests continue to promote soy as a health food. Please do your research. Start with searches on "soy" at mercola.com, or read Dr. Kaayla Daniel's groundbreaking book, *The Whole Soy Story: The Dark Side of America's Favorite Health Food*. Educating yourself is part of your wellness practice, and it's a life-long endeavor.

* * *

When you're consuming whole foods, you can easily fulfill your protein needs without putting too much thought into planning. Animal foods contain more saturated fat, so you should monitor how much you consume as well as their grades. Choose lean meats. And stick to organic milk (but only if it's already a common staple in your household). Milk is far from the "perfect" food it was once thought to be, with its allergies, intolerances, and questionable processing. On the other hand, neither is it the villain that it has been made out to be in the mainstream battle against saturated fats. A new study finds that higher milk fat intake is linked to *less* heart disease. Also to lower risk for a first heart attack. It seems that the skim milk fad may be one more health myth that we must put to bed.

---

[21] Soy products that *have* been fermented are natto, miso, tempeh, soy sauces, *fermented* tofu, and *fermented* soymilk. When used in moderation, these soy products seem to have beneficial effects on health.

When frying eggs or making omelets, use a small amount of quality coconut oil and avoid the temptation to add cheese. Coconut oil is the safest oil to use for frying since it doesn't denature as easily as other oils. Virgin olive oil is fine for cooking at lower temperatures, but not for frying temperatures. Olive oil denatures easily at frying temperatures.

And while we're on the topic of eggs, let me say this: No one, and I mean no one, has ever developed a high-cholesterol level simply by eating eggs. In fact, whole eggs contain high levels of lecithin, which reduce LDLs or bad cholesterol. Eggs are one of nature's near-perfect foods. Plus, it's hard to find another food whose proteins are more efficiently used by the body. The amino acid ratios are close to being perfect for assimilation.

So, why the bad rap for eggs? Since egg yolk is high in cholesterol, the school of thought has been that this must convert to high-cholesterol levels when digested. But it's not that simple. What goes into your mouth is not necessarily what goes into your blood. High blood cholesterol is a function of genetics, lifestyle, activity, stress, and overall diet. For example, if you totally stress out because your eggs are taken away from you, guess what will happen? Your cholesterol level will go up. But eggs do not raise cholesterol significantly, if at all. And they do not cause heart disease. In truth, they are a heart-friendly food because of their very high choline content. Choline acts like a fat solvent in the blood. And in its metabolized form, betaine, it helps protect against plaque formation in the arteries and helps clear homocysteine, a known risk factor for hardening of the arteries.

So don't freak out about eating eggs if you like them and are not allergic to them. Just don't go to excess. I often wonder why the so-called experts don't mention the other ingredients typically used in cooking eggs such as butter, grease, and lard. These substances can and will hike your cholesterol level. But do keep one thing in mind when deciding how to cook eggs: the more liquid the yolk, the healthier they are for you. Soft-boiling is the best way to cook an egg if you must. Higher temperatures that harden yolks also oxidize the cholesterol to create negative forms of LDL.

Bottom line with eggs and milk (and saturated fat in general): Plenty of data suggests that a diet high in saturated fat points to a greater risk of heart disease, especially when the diet is part of an excess-calorie regimen. So the secret for getting the benefits of eggs and milk is to eat them in moderation as part of a balance diet. Some saturated fat in the diet in the form of animal products is healthful for most people. Don't be taken in by the prevailing myths. We no longer burn people at the stake for having scurvy.

Plant proteins are an excellent source of amino acids. They just have to be combined to supply all the essentials. Without all the essential amino acids present, plant proteins will likely be digested and used for fuel instead of lean tissue development. You needn't be too concerned about this, however, unless you're a true vegetarian. As an omnivore, you seldom eat a meal strictly of fruits and vegetables. You most likely have some kind of animal protein with your meal, which supplies all the essentials. These essentials complement the incomplete amino acid sources found in your vegetables, offering additional complete protein.

If you're a vegetarian, you need to learn how to combine certain foods to form complete proteins. It's not difficult once you get the hang of it. And you don't necessarily have to eat them at the same meal, as once believed. A well-educated vegetarian can meet the necessary protein requirements to develop a nice physique while avoiding many health complications linked to the over-consumption of saturated fats found in animal products.

Protein Supplements

I've found the best daily protein intake to be between 0.6-1.25 grams for each pound of body weight. The lower third of the range is for sedentary-to-active individuals, while the higher two-thirds applies to bodybuilders and other enthusiasts pursuing lean tissue development with gusto. In any case, that's a lot of protein to get from mostly meat if you also want to moderate your meat intake. These days I seldom drink milk and typically consume eggs only 4-5 times during the week.

Up until my 38th birthday, I ate eggs nearly every morning with a tall glass of milk. I guess I got a bit burned out and decided to go the oatmeal and protein-shake route for a while. Like most people, I've developed some lactose intolerance as I've gotten older. That has induced me to limit my dairy product intake. This change has been a wise decision, as I've decreased my saturated fat intake while maintaining a healthy protein level and increasing fiber intake.

Protein supplements can be beneficial when chosen wisely. Choose only egg albumin, whey, or casein powders that contain no aspartame, sucralose, or saccharine. The latter are dangerous chemicals that *you*

121

should avoid at all costs. These chemical sweeteners lurk in such common, popular products as Nutri-Sweet®, Equal®, Splenda®, and Sweet'n Low®. A safe sweetener is stevia. You can find it in many higher quality products. Another is xylitol, when taken in smaller amounts to avoid any possible

> Aspartame, sucralose, and saccharine are dangerous chemicals you should avoid at all costs.

laxative effect. Avoid all protein bars and cookies. If you must have a treat, a protein bar would be the better choice, but these foods are mostly junk.

Here are some basics about protein supplements:

❑ Egg Protein
  ○ Has perhaps the best protein efficiency ratio, but is expensive

❑ Milk Protein
  ○ Casein: Slow digestion (time released); good before going to bed to help spare muscle during sleep
  ○ Whey: Absorbed rapidly; good following a workout. Use cross-flow, micro-filtered, or ultra-filtered products for a complete spectrum of proteins.

I usually consume one or two servings per day of a protein supplement. Supplements are much better these days, being easier to mix without using a blender. All you need is cold water and a plastic mixer found at GNC or any vitamin store. Voilà, you have an instant protein shake that's not too thick and heavy, and which tastes great.

To consume both slow- and long-acting proteins, I like to mix a scoop of vanilla whey or egg (albumin) with a scoop of banana casein. When I'm away from home, I simply pack a few scoops of protein in a plastic baggy. I also carry my shaker with me.

You may have to develop your protein supplementation level by trial and error. There are plenty of good supplements on the market, so it's hard to make a mistake. You might easily be better off buying unsweetened products and sweetening with stevia for no calories; xylitol, which has very few negatives; or more typical sweeteners such as table sugar or maple syrup, both of which are far less desirable because of their insulin-spiking effect. Still, *they don't have the more dangerous qualities of the common artificial sweeteners.* We've been finding with time that the artificial sweeteners are actually leading to more obesity (through different metabolic channels) than the old-fashioned sweeteners with calories. That's why wellness advocates must keep up-to-date with recent findings. Nutrition science is moving rapidly.

Recommended Daily Intake of Protein

- ❑ For sedentary-to-active individuals:
  - ○ 0.6 – 0.8 grams per pound of body weight
  - ○ 20% – 30% of total daily calories

- ❑ For the bodybuilder or one actively pursuing lean tissue development:
  - ○ 0.8 – 1.25 grams per pound of body weight
  - ○ 25% – 35% of total daily calories

  Note: For the bodybuilder or individual wishing to put on additional size, the percentage of daily protein calories remains fairly constant even though total calories increase.

Protein Myths

Myth 1: Excess calories from protein are used to build muscle.
Fact: Excess protein is either used as fuel or stored as fat.

Myth 2: Diets high in protein and fat, and low in carbohydrates, are best for losing weight.
Fact: These diets may be good for quick weight loss, but most of this loss is in the form of lean tissue (muscle and bone) and water. Further, these diets can actually slow your metabolism and are hard to maintain.

Myth 3: All proteins are equal.
Fact: Animal sources are superior because they contain all the essential amino acids. (Animal protein sources include supplements made from eggs, casein, and whey.)

Fat (9 calories per gram)

Without a doubt, dietary fat is the one essential that Americans are getting plenty of. The American diet is filled with saturated fat to the point that it constitutes as much as 40-50% of total calories consumed.

Combine this added "bad" fat with processed carbohydrates and you have a real health crisis on your hands. No wonder nearly two-thirds of this country's population is overweight and over thirty percent is obese. What we need is more consumption of the "good" kind of fat—unsaturated or monounsaturated. Bad fats are typically saturated and solid at room temperature, except for palm and coconut oils. Unsaturated fats include those that contain the essential fatty acids (EFAs) required in our diet.

❑ Saturated – "Bad" fats (except palm and coconut oil)
  o Animal fats
  o Some vegetable fats (vegetable shortening, margarine, cottonseed oil)
  o Solid at room temperature

❑ Unsaturated – "Good" fats containing EFAs
  o Olive, corn, sesame oils (olive is monounsaturated)
  o Nuts, fish
  o Liquid at room temperature

Fat is an essential food source because of the many roles it plays in supporting our body's health. Fat delivers energy and essential fatty acids (EFAs). It's important for our skin, hair, and nails; protects our organs from trauma; insulates our bodies; allows the transport of fat-soluble vitamins; and is needed to produce hormones and prostaglandins (cardiovascular function and inflammatory response).

Essential fatty acid deficiencies and disorders are common in the United States. Researchers think that up to 80% of the U.S. population consumes inadequate levels of EFAs. Many people don't eat food that is high in EFAs such as fish, nuts, and olive oil. Instead, they have succumbed to a diet taken directly from the pits of mass commercialization. The "pits" turns good fats into unnatural fats such as trans-fatty acids and hydrogenated fats. Altering the fat structure makes processing easier and allows food to have a longer shelf life.

Commercialized fats are void of essential fatty acids and have a negative impact on proper EFA metabolism. Most of the fats you find in processed carbohydrates are structurally altered in this way. This is one more reason to avoid boxed foods.

To make certain that my patients receive sufficient levels of EFAs in their diets, I often suggest supplementing with flax seed, fish oil, or krill oil. Flax seed oil usually comes in a liquid that should be refrigerated, while fish and krill oils are normally marketed in gel capsules (which also should be refrigerated). Keep in mind that your vitamin E intake must be sufficient if you are supplementing with EFAs. Some people do well on supplemental CLA (conjugated linoleic acid).

Aside from supplementation, you can begin enhancing your diet by changing just a few things. Use olive oil instead of vegetable oils for salads and for cooking (but not for frying). Choose cold-processed, extra virgin oil found in opaque containers, not clear bottles. Heat processing and light can denature olive oil and create "free radicals." These molecules do all kinds of damage at the least provocation, including punching holes in healthy cells.

You've heard of antioxidants? They neutralize free radicals and prevent the damaging process we commonly associate with aging. Even cooking with olive oil can denature it, so go lightly on such usage and consider using coconut oil, instead—especially for frying. Peanut oil is another option for frying because it can handle high temperatures and the fat profile is decent.

Recommended Daily Intake of Fat

For all individuals: 20% – 30% of total daily calories.

Note: When calories are restricted, the total percentage of fat in the diet may increase because of a reduction in carbohydrates. The same is true of the protein percentage. Yet, the *grams* of protein required per pound of body weight must remain about the same.

Fat Myths

Myth 1: As long as my carbohydrate intake is low, it's okay to consume a moderate, high-fat diet.

Fact: The typical American high-fat diet is always unhealthy and can increase your risk of cardiovascular disease. This is a diet high in omega 6's with too many animal fats, polyunsaturated fats, hydrogenated fats, and transfats.

Myth 2: You must cut out all fat when trying to lose weight.

Fact: Omega-3 and omega-6 fatty acids are essential for fat metabolism. This means monounsaturated, polyunsaturated, and saturated fats from coconut oil are essential. However, *too many polyunsaturated fats can create a poor omega-3 to omega-6 ratio.*

Fact: Fats play a critical role in our overall health, from hormone syntheses to the transport of fat-soluble vitamins.

Fact: Fats aid in satiety and prevent overeating.

Fact: Moderate, high-fat diets (high in omega 3's) are okay and can be valuable for minimizing fat-storing hormones like insulin.

Water (0 calories per gram)

Yes, water is one of the essentials we can't forget about. It makes up 50%–70% of our body weight and 65%–75% of our lean body weight. Hydrating your body should become a top priority if it isn't already.

Dehydration places stress on the entire body and hampers normal metabolic processes. Preventing dehydration means ingesting fluids intermittently throughout the entire day, whether you get them from certain foods (fruits and vegetables) or from liquids. If you're one who maintains a diet high in fruits and vegetables, you are less vulnerable to the effects of dehydration. Overall, the majority of us need to pay extra attention to the amount of water we consume and make a conscious effort to drink it whenever we get the chance. Water is the nutrient that bathes our cells and provides a medium for the chemical reactions that support life.

If you don't already have one, lease a bottled-water dispenser (the 5-gallon type) or consider a good filter system (probably reverse osmosis) that also removes fluoride if it's being added to your water supply. I highly recommend it. Since my wife and I had a bottled-water system placed in our home, I find myself drinking more just because it's cold, convenient, and good. No need for ice or keeping pitchers filled for refrigeration. Just grab a glass or shaker and fill it up. Making my protein drinks is a snap. It also saves money compared to purchasing cases of the individual bottles. Anytime we wish to take water with us, we just fill up an empty bottle or two and we're good to go.

Besides the unseen miracles that water constantly provides within and around our cells, it also provides visible changes. Being well-hydrated offers your skin its best chance of looking full and youthful beyond what any "state of the art" cosmetics claim to be capable of doing. And once

126

you begin to develop that well-toned body, your adequate hydration level keeps your muscles full and skin taut. So drink up!

Recommended Daily Intake of Water

Instead of other less desirable substitutes, drink water when you are thirsty. If you're choosing water as your main source of fluids, you don't need to worry about how many glasses or ounces you consume each day. Trying to drink gallons of water a day in no way adds additional benefits to your health regimen. In fact, this can actually disrupt the normal potassium and sodium balance in your cells. When such disruption occurs, you find yourself retaining fluids because potassium is being lost.

By the way, as you get older, your sense of thirst may diminish and you may find yourself taking insufficient water. Yet, if you've been paying attention to your water needs over time, this is unlikely to happen because you are more attuned to your "real" thirst.

More on Food and Nutritional Supplements

Building a great body comes not from dietary supplements, but primarily from resistance training and eating nutritious meals. Yes, certain supplements can help. But, by definition, their job is only to "supplement" the diet so that there is little risk of missing key components that could hinder development. They do not substitute for nutritious foods.

I don't believe in miracle pills or powders and therefore have never placed too much emphasis on finding shortcuts to proper diet and training. As I mentioned earlier, however, a good protein supplement may be necessary if one is to consume the necessary daily amount of that nutrient. Here is a list of supplements that should be a part of your diet:

- ❏ Protein powder (milk, whey, casein)
  - o Provides an excellent source of amino acids that deliver complete protein
  - o Is essential for lean tissue growth

- ❏ Essential fatty acids (flaxseed, fish, krill oils, CLA [conjugated linoleic acid])
  - o Are essential for cardiovascular health and endocrine (hormone) function

- o   Provide phytoestrogens that help balance the ratio of estrogen to progesterone
- o   Are required for fat metabolism (fat burning)
- o   Help to minimize or reduce hidden inflammation in conditions such as fibromyalgia and lupus

❑   Vitamin / mineral supplementation
- o   Because the American diet is deficient of key nutrients
- o   Because you can find companies that have a proven track record and scientific research to back up the efficiency of their products. Pharmaceutical-grade products are best because of quality and quantity consistency.

❑   Antioxidants
- o   Often called anti-aging chemicals, these act as scavengers and bind up free radicals that cause cellular damage.

Antioxidants

You need to protect yourself from the harmful effects of free radicals that I mentioned under the discussion on fats. Pollutants in the air we breathe, poor living habits, and oils and fats heated to high temperatures are just a few sources of these damaging molecules.

Many of today's scientists believe free radicals are one of the primary causes of aging. Free radicals create cellular damage that can lead to common conditions found in the middle-aged and elderly such as arteriosclerosis and skin damage. It's also known that certain chemicals or compounds found in fruits and vegetables offer a solution to controlling or minimizing the negative effects of free radicals. These fruit and vegetable compounds can be extracted and concentrated in the form of dietary supplements that let us achieve adequate ingestion in antioxidant-deficient diets. I regularly supplement my diet with good vitamins and minerals as well as antioxidants. Common antioxidants are alpha lipoic acid, co-enzyme Q10, l-taurine, glutathionine, vitamins C & E, and selenium. Green tea, fruits, vegetables, and often their abstracts, are also good natural sources of antioxidants. By the way, virtually all overweight people are low in antioxidants.[22]

---

[22] Richards, Byron J., with Mary Guignon Richards, *Mastering Leptin: Your Guide to Permanent Weight Loss and Permanent Health,* Third Edition, Wellness Resources Books, ISBN 978-1-933927-21-1, p. 91.

Anti-Inflammation Joint Support

I began noticing "calendar" effects at about 35. It was subtle at first—just slight joint discomfort upon waking and a few "crow lines" appearing at the corners of my eyes. No matter how well we seem to take care of ourselves, the effects of time show up eventually because of inevitable stress buildup.

I knew I had been pretty hard on myself growing up, participating in year-round sports, choosing outdoor physical work such as home construction instead of desk work, and enjoying the sun to its fullest. This lifestyle continued throughout my undergraduate years up until my entrance into post-graduate school to earn my doctorate.

Although the outdoor jobs stopped, I remained physically engaged both in my career as a chiropractor and in maintaining my physique. If you've ever visited a chiropractor, you understand the vigorous physical demands required of this profession. After 16 years of practice, I needed a break. My neck, lower back, and wrists were telling me that something had to change.

Obviously, cutting down on the volume of my patients was the first step in diminishing the day-to-day stress on my joints. But I needed something more and certainly wanted to avoid the detrimental effects of non-steroidal anti-inflammatory drugs (NSAIDS). I eventually began supplementing with glucosamine and chondroitin sulfate. Although these non-prescription aids offered no *immediate* relief, I began to notice a lessening of my symptoms over time. These substances act on the hyaline cartilage to repair and maintain it, while simultaneously aiding in the anti-inflammatory process. Another similarly acting substance is gamma-linolenic acid, or GLA. It's a fatty acid found primarily in vegetable oils.

You also have many other opportunities available to you in the form of anti-inflammatory herbs. After all, you're much better off protecting yourself and *preventing* the eroding effects of chronic joint inflammation than attempting to fix and repair damage after the fact. Here's a list of the most common anti-inflammatory herbs. Notice that many are used in cooking recipes:

Tumeric, ginger, boswellia, curcumin, capsaicin, green tea, oregano, holy basil, rosemary, licorice, autumn saffron, German chamomile, bromelain, arnica, hu zhang, Chinese

goldthread, Chinese barberry, scutellaria, pokeroot, cleavers, devil's claw, white willow, and witch hazel.

A non-prescription supplement called Zyflamend and Zyflamend PM (products of New Chapter, Inc.) are also reported to be getting good results. The first contains 10 herbs, nine from the above list. Actually, there are many herbal formulas on the market that may help. Wellness-oriented people look for the best and are willing to experiment because individual needs vary. Also, there's a lot of hype out there that we have to work through or unmask.

Finally, in terms of regular dietary measures, the following will help you reduce inflammation:

Eliminate polyunsaturated vegetable oils, margarine, vegetable shortening, all partially hydrogenated oils, and all foods that contain trans-fatty acids (read food labels to check for the presence of these oils). Instead, use extra-virgin olive oil as your main fat (except when cooking at high temperatures, where coconut oil is better), and increase your intake of omega-3 fatty acids found in walnuts, oily, cold-water fish, flaxseeds or flax oil and fish oil and krill oil supplements.

A Brief Note about Fanaticism

One can devote an *incredible* amount of attention to nutrition, and some people do exactly that in the hopes that it will solve all their sickness problems. At the end of the day, however, a wellness-oriented person looks to see how life connects in *all* its fascinating ways. Becoming a nutrition fanatic at the expense of the many other opportunities for wellness practice won't get the job done. For example, it's good to remember that the junk coming out of our mouths may make us just as sick as any junk that goes in. Usually more so.

12: Launching Your 12-Week Nutrition Plan

You now have the basic information and know what you should and shouldn't eat as well as how often. The question now is, Are you ready to take the steps required to change your present eating habits into the habits of champions? I hope you can now answer with an emphatic, *yes*. This is the most important part of the program when it comes to shedding body fat and improving your overall health.

> **Resistance training becomes effective only with proper and adequate nutrition. If you fail at this, I can guarantee you'll fail at achieving your ultimate goal of body metamorphosis.**

Whenever I'm feeling less than optimal and my muscles are a bit flat, I can always trace the problem to my recent diet. For me, it usually means I've been skipping meals. I make the adjustment and, within two or three days, I begin to feel and see positive changes. It never fails.

Chances are you need to make decisions on how to handle some of the processed foods currently occupying space in your kitchen cabinets, refrigerator, and freezer. This can be difficult, especially if you have younger children who are used to having treats when they get home from school. So what do you do?

One can hope your children are open to the idea of eating a more healthful diet. However, you're in charge of making the decisions that affect the health of your children. This doesn't mean you have to immediately throw the Cap'n Crunch and the Oreo cookies into the garbage. However, you will need to slowly make changes in the foods you purchase. If your kids run the palace, then a permanent change in your eating habits and those of your children will be hard if not impossible to come by. Poorer health and obesity will be everyone's lot.

Start by replacing high sugar and fat foods with a variety of healthy snacks such as naturally sweetened whole grain treats, fruits, and nuts. I say this to help you make the needed adjustments. Most artificial sweeteners and unnatural fats have health risks of their own. Within a few weeks you should be able to clean out most of the bad stuff without creating a major family crisis. And you do have to become a detective if you want wellness for your family.

131

For example, recent TV promotions for Nutella® tout it to be some kind of healthy spread. But the ads mislead! The two most prevalent Nutella ingredients are sugar and fat, in that order. Fifty percent of the calories come from fat and 40% from sugar. How healthy is that? If you put it on bread, you have a piece of bread with an unhealthy spread!

So how do you shop for the good stuff? The same way you shop for the bad: just change the foods you are putting into your cart. Go to the *Reclaim 24* Food Guide in Appendix B and choose foods from each category. If you follow this, you can't make many mistakes on what you bring home. My wife and I rarely purchase treats except for some occasional graham crackers and whipped cream. I'm better off not having "treats" around the house. Out of sight, out of mind. When we feel like having a treat, we have to go out to get it. This system works like that used by our hunter-gatherer ancestors. If they wanted it, they had to go out to get it! More often than not, I won't bother.

If you must have some of the bad stuff around, don't sweat it too much. You'll slowly find that as your leptin metabolism get balanced, you will have little craving for treats. Take it a step at a time.

The "Joys" of Calorie Counting

To begin your 12-week program, you first need to know approximately how many calories you're consuming and how many you *should be* consuming. As a doctor, I've learned the value of objectivity. This means having a way to realistically measure where you are at your starting point (your baseline) as well as a way to measure the changes that follow.

Please don't get carried away with calorie counting. However, if you don't know what your present baseline number is, you'll fail to understand how this correlates to your present dietary habits. Do you even have an idea how many calories you consume in a day? Chances are you don't. It's important to be aware of your daily calorie consumption once you start your 12-week program because you may see the need to adjust your calories upward or downward.

The body frequently tricks us into thinking it needs the opposite of what it actually does. I often see men and women working hard at the gym and making a gallant effort with their diets. They see weight come off, but what they don't see is much change in body tone or hardness. They are really just becoming physically shrunken versions of what they were, but the soft parts are still there—where they don't want them to be.

Strange as it seems, do you know what most of them do when that happens? They cut their calories back even further and work harder and longer at the gym. <u>But that is a mistake</u>. When they do this, the body eats its own lean tissue for energy, lowering the person's body weight without a positive change in muscle tone. You can avoid this mistake if you know the number of calories you're now ingesting and the number you're supposed to be ingesting to achieve your purpose.

You would think that someone who is already losing weight would rule out further reductions in caloric intake while trying to get toned. But I've witnessed time after time that they do not rule it out. They're waiting for some magical change to occur in their muscle tone by eating less. Again, the body can trick our minds. Or equally destructive, we listen to misinformed people.

Look at page 134 to view the tables included the **Daily Calorie Requirements Guide**. I've designed these simplified tables to help you quickly calculate the number of calories you need to consume each day to lose fat, maintain weight, or grow muscle—all based on your current body composition and activity level.

You need to estimate how much you exceed your ideal weight by identifying your body fat percentage. One of the best ways to do this is with calipers. If you don't have access to calipers or other devices that can help you pinpoint your body fat percentage *and what that means in terms of excess pounds*, you can always estimate your ideal body weight from your high-school days. If you were unhappy with your shape even then, get your body fat tested or invest in some calipers.

Once you've identified how much fat you need to shed to get your body fat percentage where you want it, you'll know which table to use. Then you identify your activity level and find the appropriate cell in the table based on whether you want to lose fat, maintain the status quo, or grow muscle. Multiply the number in the cell with your current body weight to get your required daily calories. If you're going to jump right into the *Reclaim 24* body-shaping workout, then you need to judge yourself as being at least "active"—maybe "very active."

Okay, you will find the Calorie Requirements Guide on the next page. Following that are three quick examples of how someone would calculate the required calories for their level of overweight, their level of physical activity, and their body-change goal.

Daily Calorie Requirements Guide

Sedentary–Minimal activity at work and no regular exercise program.

Active–May or may not have physically demanding job, but routinely involved in physical activities such as bicycling or intermittent exercise.

Very Active–Involved in a very active lifestyle that includes a regular weight resistance exercise program and/or sports.

Note–Men must add 1 point to any cell multiplier number when calculating the calories required.

15 lbs. *or less* overweight

	Lose	Maintain	Grow
Sedentary	11 x Body Wt	13 x Body Wt	15 x Body Wt
Active	12 x Body Wt	14 x Body Wt	16 x Body Wt
Very Active	13 x Body Wt	15 x Body Wt	17 x Body Wt

16 – 25 lbs. Overweight

	Lose	Maintain
Sedentary	10 x Body Wt	12 x Body Wt
Active	11 x Body Wt	13 x Body Wt
Very Active	12 x Body Wt	14 x Body Wt

All Cell Multiplier Numbers in the three tables are for Women. Men must add 1 to each cell number.

26 – 40 lbs. Overweight (*Maximum caloric intake not to exceed 2,400 no matter what the calculation*)

	Lose	Maintain
Sedentary	8 x Body Wt	10 x Body Wt
Active	9 x Body Wt	11 x Body Wt
Very Active	10 x Body Wt	12 x Body Wt

41 lb or more: Subtract 15 % from total calories computed *using the 26-40 lb. table.* After dropping below 41 lbs., follow the 26-40 lb. guidelines, making sure you restrict total calories to 2400—no matter what the calculation—any time you are 26 or more pounds overweight.

Some sample calculations follow that show how to use the Guide:

1. Active *female* weighing 165 lbs. and approximately 25 lbs. overweight (use 2nd table) and wanting to lose fat:

   Number of daily calories needed to lose weight = 11 x 165 or <u>1,815</u> total daily calories

2. Very active *male* weighing 184 lbs. and 0 lbs. overweight (use 1st table) and wishing to grow muscle:

   Number of daily calories needed to grow muscle = 184 x 18 or <u>3,312</u> total daily calories (remembering to add 1 to the cell number for men)

3. Active *female* weighing 179 lbs. and about 40 lbs. overweight (use 3rd table) and wanting to lose fat:

   Number of daily calories needed to lose weight = 179 x 9 or <u>1,611</u> total daily calories

4. Active *male* weighing 260 pounds and 45 pounds overweight (look below 3rd table) and wanting to lose fat:

   Number of daily calories needed to lose weight = 260 x 10 or <u>2600</u> total calories. But <u>he must now subtract 15%</u> of that number as long as he remains 41 pounds or more overweight. This reduces to <u>2210</u> daily calories for the time being.

Notice how the table values grow smaller as the overweight categories grow larger (top-down in the tables). This says that the more fat that you have present, the fewer calories you need to support each pound of body weight. *That's because muscle requires many more calories for 24/7 maintenance than do stores of fat.*

As you can see from the Guide, you need to alter your calories as you begin to achieve your goals, shifting from one table to another and from the "lose" or "grow" columns to the "maintain" column.

> **If you have been following the latest fad diets, you may initially think that the daily calorie values cited in the Calorie Requirements Guide are a little high. The reason for this confusion is that "experts" in the field of *self-cannibalism* design those fad diets!**

That's right, cannibalism. If you wish to lose weight really, really fast because you have a swim party to attend next week, then the quickest way to shed that weight is to dehydrate yourself, remove normal intestinal sludge, burn up some of your unwanted muscle, a little unwanted bone tissue, and maybe even a smidgen of fat. Do you think you're carrying excess water? That's a myth. Either you're carrying too much fat or you're not. Water isn't the villain obscuring your "six-pack" abs. If your goal is to lose body fat while growing muscle, you must trust me on this one. Losing body fat while maintaining or growing muscle isn't a process you can rush for next week's swim party! Quick weight loss is not healthy, it's not attractive, and it won't last. Repeat: *It's not healthy, it's not attractive, and it won't last!*

Remember, the calories you consume are good calories dispersed over three meals (more only by exception) a day, including breakfast. This makes for an efficient energy metabolism. With the right nutrient mixture, meal timing and calories, your body realizes that it's not in starvation mode, so it burns calories normally to give you the energy you need. Diets that restrict your calories too much only result in a crash-and-burn process, leaving you confused, depressed, and less healthy. The swim party simply isn't worth it. Wear clothes or skip it altogether.

Once you've identified your caloric starting point with the Daily Calorie Requirements Guide, you next need to *copy* the **Reclaim 24 Daily Nutrition Track Sheet.** You can find this track sheet on the two pages starting at page 138. You want to make multiple copies of the two pages for recording your daily food intake. You'll may also download a more convenient copy of the track sheet from my overall wellness website, **www.drcharleswebb.com**.

The track sheet helps you record your daily intake of protein, carbohydrates, fat, and total calories. At the end of each day, you are able to quickly identify what's out of balance and make adjustments for the next day. After doing this for a few days, you don't need to complete the track sheet every day because you'll know from the foods you're eating whether you're in the ballpark. You will, however, need to return to charting for a couple of days *at the beginning of each month* when you recalculate your caloric needs because of a change in weight, activity level, and maybe even your goal (lose, maintain, grow).

Many authors suggest that calorie counting only results in failure because it ultimately drives a counter crazy and places too many demands on him or her. I agree—that is if calorie counting becomes a persistent part of your life. On the other hand, when a need for calorie adjustments arises, you must use objective markers to make educated decisions on what to do next. Flying by the seat of your pants will not work. Many have tried. All but the luckiest have failed.

Some authors suggest the "deck of playing cards" or "palm size" rule to keep calorie intake in its optimum range. This means your portion size should fit in the palm of your hand—about the volume of a deck of playing cards. This isn't a bad approach. It certainly helps those who suffer from the "fork to mouth" syndrome, but it also fails to address several factors. For example, my wife weighs 108 lbs. I weigh around 200. I should be consuming at least 65–80% more calories than she. If we both eat portions the size of a deck of playing cards, one or both of us will be changing our body composition in unhealthy ways.

With time—and certainly once you've reached your goals—counting calories will no longer be necessary. Your body and eating habits will tell you when you need to kick the calories up or bring them down. You can usually accomplish this by altering particular foods in your diet. Never reduce caloric intake by skipping meals. NEVER! *Your body goes into starvation mode!* The next thing you know you'll have fat in places you don't want it and your energy levels will dive, making it difficult or impossible to build muscle or enjoy life. Don't skip meals. This means breakfast, too. This is one more place where your self-discipline is essential. Again, it's about replacing bad habits with good ones.

Today's the Day!

First, determine your present dietary habits as best you can. Use the **Reclaim 24 Food Guide** at Appendix B to help you measure, on a daily basis, your present caloric intake as well as the protein, carbohydrate, and fat content of your diet. Working with the numbers in the Food Guide, you are able to complete your Daily Nutrition Track Sheet using a *copy* of the track sheet on the two pages starting at page 138. You then average your caloric and nutrient intake over the course of at least three days to get reliable numbers.

Also, note the frequency and times of your meals. Your new eating lifestyle requires that you consume your three regular meals, breakfast, lunch, and dinner. Yes, breakfast, too. If you can't find the majority of your foods within the Food Guide to do your calculations, *you're probably eating too much junk.* Many of the fast-food chains offer nutrition guides, so I suggest picking them up at future visits.

Reclaim 24 Daily Nutrition Track Sheet

Breakfast

	Calories	Protein (g)	Carbs (g)	Fat (g)
Breakfast Subtotals→				

Lunch

	Calories	Protein (g)	Carbs (g)	Fat (g)
Lunch Subtotals→				

Optional Meal*

	Calories	Protein (g)	Carbs (g)	Fat (g)
Optional Subtotals→				

*This optional meal is not a part of the normal *Reclaim 24* eating plan, but for those making a transition to three standard meals per day. It is also for those who are especially active and who need the extra meal and calories.

Dinner¤	Calories¤	Protein (g)¤	Carbs (g)¤	Fat (g)¤
¤	¤	¤	¤	¤
¤	¤	¤	¤	¤
¤	¤	¤	¤	¤
¤	¤	¤	¤	¤
¤	¤	¤	¤	¤
Dinner Subtotals →¤	¤	¤	¤	¤
¤	¤	¤	¤	¤
Add Meal Subtotals for Breakfast, Lunch Dinner, And "Optional" (if used) ¤	A:¤	B:¤	C:¤	D:¤
Calculate the three formulas to get your nutrient percentages for the entire day and enter them here ¤		(Bx400)÷A¤	(Cx400)÷A¤	(Dx900)÷A¤
		¤	¤	¤

Instructions: 1. For each of the three (optionally four) meals, list the foods eaten along with their calorie and nutrient numbers as found in the *Reclaim 24 Food Guide* of Appendix B. ¶

2. Add up the four columns under each meal and place the sums in the subtotal blocks for those meals. ¶

3. Add up the three (or four) meal *subtotals* and enter the sums into blocks A, B, C and D. ¶

4. Use the formulas shown to compute the daily percentages for each nutrient. For example, in the first formula calculation block, multiply the value of block B by 400 then divide by the value in block A. ¶

This track sheet may also be found at www.reclaim24.com for your convenience in printing. ¶

139

Day Planning

Plan and track your calorie counting by filling out copies of the *Reclaim 24* Daily Nutrition Track Sheet. You already know how many calories you should be ingesting because you calculated the number using the Daily Calorie Requirements Guide on page 134. Your track sheets will help you understand how close you are to that calorie target. In addition, you are able to see how close your protein, carbohydrate, and fat intakes are relative to the percentage intervals recommended for your goal. From Chapter 11 (*The Nutrients and Other Dietary Essentials*), here's a <u>recommendations summary</u> for each nutrient:

Carbohydrates

To grow muscle:
   55-65% *of total calories*

To maintain weight:
   50-55% *of total calories*

To lose weight (fat)
   40-50% *of total calories*

Proteins

For the sedentary or active individual:
   0.6 – 0.8 grams per pound of body weight
   20% – 30% of total daily calories

For the bodybuilder or one actively pursuing lean tissue development:
   0.8 – 1.25 grams per pound of body weight
   25% – 35% of total daily calories

Fats

For all activity levels, 20% - 30% of total daily calories

Let's now recap. So far you know two things: (1) how many *calories* you should be consuming each day to meet your chosen goal of "lose," "maintain," or "grow," and (2) what *percentages* of those daily calories should be taken up by *carbohydrates, proteins,* and *fats.*

Next, you convert those three percentages into *grams* so that you know what your *target* grams for each nutrient should be to achieve your goal. Finally, on a Daily Nutrition Track Sheet, you record your *actual* daily intake of each nutrient in grams. Once done, you may compare your calculated *target* grams for the three nutrients with your *actual* grams of consumption. You then make future adjustments as needed.

Okay, that explains what we're trying to do. Now here's an example to show you how you should go about calculating your target grams of carbohydrates, proteins, and fats.

For this example, Tracy, an <u>active female</u>, weighs <u>154 pounds,</u> and wants to <u>lose about 20 pounds of fat</u>. She will now step through her calculations.

1. **Calculating Tracy's Daily Calorie Target:** Looking at the Calorie Requirements Guide on page 134[23], Tracy sees that the number of calories she needs to consume each day is 154 x 11 = <u>1,694 calories</u>.

2. **Calculating Tracy's Daily Carbohydrate Target in Grams:** From the nutrients summary on page 140, Tracy sees her carbohydrate target to be 40%-50% of her total calories. She chooses the high number of the range, 50%[24] or one-half. That makes Tracy's carbohydrate target 847 calories (1694 ÷ 2). But how many *grams* of carbohydrates does that amount to? 847 ÷ 4[25] = 211.75 grams, or <u>212 grams</u> rounded off.

3. **Calculating Tracy's Daily Protein Target in Grams:** As seen in the recommendations summary on page 140, two computations are in order for the <u>active</u> individual: grams per pound of bodyweight

---

[23] She uses the *second* table in the guide (16–25 lbs.) because it applies to her 20-lb weight-loss goal.

[24] Seldom will you need to ingest less than 50% in carbohydrates, but you may drop them down as low as 40% for short periods. Carbohydrate intake of less than 50% of total calories will mostly be restricted to those who are extremely overweight and/or who have *insulin resistance* (detailed in Chapter 14, "The Role of Hormones in Wellness"). As you lose weight, your overall caloric intake will need a boost—mostly in the form of complex carbohydrates—pushing the overall percentage of carbohydrates closer to the 55% mark.

[25] You learned in Chapter 11 that carbohydrates contain 4 calories per gram. Therefore, we divide 847 calories by 4 to see what Tracy's daily carbohydrate target should be in grams.

and percentage of total calories. First, to get grams per pound of bodyweight, Tracy adopts the middle figure, 0.7, of the target range, 0.6 – 0.8. She then multiplies 0.7 by her body weight, 154, and gets 107.8 grams. She rounds that off to 108 grams of protein.

The second computation is the percentage of total calories that protein should represent in her diet. Again Tracy picks the middle of the protein range for the active person (20% – 30%), and that is 25%. So her daily protein target in calories is 423.5, which is 25% of her total daily calories of 1,694. But how many *grams* of protein is that? Recalling from Chapter 11 that each gram of protein, like carbohydrates, is equivalent to 4 calories, she divides 423.5 by 4 to get 105.875 grams of protein. Round that off to 106 grams.

So Tracy now has two numbers to represent her daily protein target: 108 and 106. She takes the average to get <u>107 grams</u>.

4. **Calculating Tracy's Daily Fat Target in Grams:** Again, looking at the nutrients summary on page 140, Tracy sees that her daily target for fat calories should be 20% – 30% of her total. Keeping in mind that she has already targeted about 1,271 calories of 1,694 for carbohydrates and proteins (847 + 423.5), she's left with 423 calories for fat intake. Does this fit the target range of 20% – 30%? We can find out by dividing the 423 fat calories by the daily total of 1694. We get 24.9%, which we can round off to 25%. That certainly falls within the fat-target range of 20% – 30%, so Tracy is on firm ground (you're welcome to entertain a pun here).

The next thing she needs to do is convert the fat calories to grams of fat. Again, remembering from Chapter 11 that one gram of fat contains 9 calories (rather than the 4 calories contained in a gram of carbohydrates or protein), she divides the 423 calories by 9 to get her daily fat target of <u>47 grams</u>.

So there we have it. Tracy now knows what her objective targets are in terms of daily calories and nutrients: 1,694 calories composed of 212 grams of carbohydrate, 107 grams of protein, and 47 grams of fat. Always remember that you need to convert between calories and grams by the using the equivalents of 4 calories per gram for carbohydrates and proteins, and 9 calories per gram for fats.

Now Tracy can begin filling out her Daily Nutrition Track Sheet using values she finds in the Appendix B Food Guide. In this way, she discovers what she is *really* consuming and starts to modify her food intake to make sure her body-renewal diet gets much closer to the targets she computed for herself.

You needn't be overly concerned if you find your percentages to be off-target after calculating them at the end of the day. Make small adjustments with the types of foods you eat until the numbers get closer to the computed targets (which follow the guidelines on page 140).

Using the Daily Nutrition Track Sheet as a tool for planning and tracking helps you stay in the ballpark without forcing you to scientifically analyze every meal you eat. Some days you'll be right on the money, and some days a little bit off. It won't matter. Overall, this tool helps you learn how to make conscious decisions in your food choices and become more intuitive about nutrient mixes so you soon don't have to think about it so much that your head hurts.

It's funny how the simple process of tracking what we eat keeps us from making unwise choices. I guess it's easier to *pretend* we're eating right when we don't have to see a noontime brownie written down anywhere. Out of sight, out of mind. And no conscious guilt! Believe me, this Track Sheet exercise will help you with your discipline.

Once you have some control over your eating habits, feel free to throw the track sheets away. And enjoy the pool party coming up in a few months!

Meal Planning

If you're a planning person then I highly suggest you carry that trait over to your meal planning. I'm not a planner and therefore rarely plan my meals, or any non-work related activity for that matter. I'm more spur-of-the-moment and decide what's going into my mouth about 20 minutes before mealtime. Because of who I am, this simplifies my life. The main goal is to make certain that you eat three complete meals with the proper distances between them. Your meals should consist of protein, vegetables, grain/starch, and/or fruit. You can also make individual meals (breakfast, for example) using a small portion of non-salted nuts, a piece of fruit, and a protein supplement. Protein supplements allow for simplicity and help you save time, especially while working. But no meal skipping!

As a neat trick to keep you on the right dietary path, try consuming two or three organically grown apples each day. The apple's fructose (in the whole-fruit form) satisfies your sugar cravings while the pectin (soluble fiber) helps suppress your appetite. *Fructose added to the diet in its processed, concentrated forms (e.g., high-fructose corn syrup, fruit juice, fructose crystals) is <u>not</u> healthful, no matter what the advertisers say!*

So here's your summary:

- ❏ Eat three complete meals (and a fourth is absolutely necessary):
  - ○ Include protein, vegetables, grain/starch, and occasional fruit.
  - ○ Never skip breakfast!

- ❏ At times, meals can consist of:
  - ○ A protein supplement that can easily be mixed with water
  - ○ A palmful of unsalted nuts—almonds, cashews, pecans, and walnuts supply energy and *suppress appetite*
  - ○ Fruit or small salad

Maintaining a Healthy Energy Metabolism

When you follow the *Reclaim 24* program as I've outlined it, you will foster a "non-starvation" energy metabolism. The key to this is eating smartly and never skipping meals. That *is* simple, isn't it?

And guess what else helps to keep your metabolic furnace and energy levels stoked? Remember the "cheat day" I mentioned in Chapter 10? The cheat day allows you to consume up to an additional 20-25% more calories in a single day of whatever foods you crave. Cravings that come from metabolic imbalances don't go away overnight, but they *will* go away if you stay with this program. You're better off cheating just a little bit every four or five days and staying with the program than playing the part of a martyr and suddenly crashing and burning. That's what happens to most people who try to deprive themselves using willpower. Their willpower just gets bowled over because their hormonal cravings are irrepressible. Then these folks binge for days or weeks at a time in the worst possible ways. Back to ground zero—or worse.

Back to cheating. Your body needs to be shaken up now and then so it doesn't adapt to the same old things (the body just loves to adapt). If your calories are mildly restricted over time, your body may start slowing things down to protect itself from starvation (more homeostasis in action). By giving your system some extra fuel periodically, you can avoid this protective reaction altogether.

Periodically means every four or five days. Every fourth or fifth day you get to "fall off the wagon" and treat yourself to whatever it is that stimulates your taste buds. But this isn't a free pass to go crazy! Twenty-five percent of a 2,500-calorie diet is an additional 625 calories, or a few hundred shy of that "Super Size" meal. Furthermore, *a cheat day doesn't mean you must consume the extra calories in the form of junk.* You may also enjoy just eating more *good* food. As you get closer to achieving your fitness and weight goals, you'll find that you can cheat a bit more often. But make no mistake about it: "cheating" may slow down your fat burning for a day or two since the extra metabolic boost that comes from surprising the body may not fully cover the extra calories consumed. And it may temporarily affect your leptin metabolism. Nonetheless, once you've reached your desired levels of fitness and fat reduction, don't be afraid to cheat four or five times a week, just so long as you continue to work hard, you experience *real* hunger once or twice a day (especially in the morning), and you keep your overall diet clean.

Update Your Caloric Requirements in Four-Week Cycles

If you are on the "lose" program, you also avoid a slowdown of your metabolism by updating your daily caloric requirements and your cheat-day allowance every four weeks. Of course, you do these calculations at the beginning of your first four weeks when you start your program (as Tracy did beginning on page 141). Then you calculate again at the beginning of weeks 5–8, and again at the beginning of weeks 9–12.

You use the appropriate table from the Calorie Requirements Guide according to your weight and the number of pounds you need to lose at the beginning of the cycle. You also calculate 20%–25% of your calorie allowance so that you know what your cheat-day allowance should be. Remember, both your calorie requirements and cheat allowance will change each cycle because you are losing weight. But you can still cheat every fourth or fifth day according to the allowance in effect at the time.

At the End of 12-Weeks

At the end of your 12-week program, you should have certainly changed your physique for the better—much better. Don't be overly concerned with your body weight as much as the change in your appearance. If you follow my program correctly, you'll be shedding body fat while adding lean tissue. Muscle and other lean tissue are more

145

dense than fat. They take up less room, actually a lot less room. This means you become a smaller, firmer you even if your weight doesn't change. So don't worry about your final weight as long as your body looks like the one you want to wear!

And once the 12-week metamorphosis is complete, don't think you can just quit and take it easy. You must continue to nurture it as long as you are breathing. Please note that this is not a diet or weight-loss program we're talking about here: *Reclaim 24* is a lifestyle! Diets and weight-loss programs are temporary and seldom healthy or worth the effort. Lifestyle changes—the proper lifestyle changes, that is—are not temporary and are definitely worth the effort. The good news is that it takes only half as much effort to maintain your new body as it took to create it.

But what do you do after 12 weeks if you are not seeing the results you want? What if desperation is beginning to set in?

On rare occasions, a person who diligently follows the 12-week *Reclaim 24* Action Plan is not able to lose fat or gain muscle. Such people most likely have worked with discipline at other programs but have been unable to shed stubborn fat or change their appearance very much. If you're among them, almost surely your hormones, lifestyle, or both are too far out of balance to handle yourself. In other words, you're still not truly "well," despite your diet and exercise efforts, despite your efforts at setting aside old habits, and despite the best use of your imagination. Some may think you lack discipline—but you know better! Yet, without progress, you can easily get desperate, run off in many directions at the same time, and make some serious blunders.

In my practice I offer an offsite program to help folks like you receive the *personally tailored* information they need to understand what's going on with their health. Also, to understand the action plan they must adopt to overcome their stubborn weight-loss problem. But because you may not have access to my boot camp, **in the next chapter, I run through the important points you must understand about your challenge if you are not getting the results you want.** But first, to close this chapter, here are some frequently asked questions that I get on nutrition, along with answers.

146

Frequently Asked Questions

Q: There's so much confusion concerning carbohydrates. Many diets today tell us to eat more fat and protein and minimize carbohydrate consumption. Are carbs really that bad for us?

A: Absolutely not. In fact, carbohydrates are our body's preferred energy source. As well, they are essential for burning fat properly. Without enough carbohydrates in our diet, our body begins to use protein for fuel, resulting in muscle and bone loss. With the loss of lean tissue, our overall metabolism slows down causing our bodies to store additional fat. Carbohydrates, *in their more natural state,* also provide fiber for our digestive tract, allowing excess cholesterol and other wastes to be bound and carried out of our system. In the form of fruits and high-fiber vegetables, carbohydrates supply vital nutrients and antioxidants not found in animal sources.

Q: Simple sugar is a carbohydrate, so why is it so bad for you?

A: Not all carbohydrates are equal when it comes to the overall health of your body. When you ingest carbohydrates, your blood sugar rises. In response to this, your pancreas produces insulin. Insulin is a hormone that transports blood sugar (glucose) into the body's cells. Complex carbohydrates, such as vegetables and most whole grains, cause a slower rise in blood sugar, allowing the pancreas a longer period to control this transportation process. Simple sugars cause a sudden and rapid rise in blood sugar levels. This stresses the pancreas. With day-in and day-out ingestion of these simple sugars—often a large portion of processed foods—the continued stress on the pancreas can lead to its loss of full function. Also, high levels of continuous insulin secretion create insulin resistance in the very cells that need insulin for effective nourishment.

Here's how things work. When we experience hunger or low energy, the first thing we think of is carbohydrates. This is because our body recognizes carbs as providing a fast cure for hunger. In a healthy system, insulin is produced following the smallest ingestion of food. This helps to pass blood sugar into the needy cells and also to prevent blood sugar levels from getting too high (which is dangerous). Then, once sugar enters the cells, a satiation signal is sent to the brain to turn off hunger. So we stop eating, blood sugar levels return to normal, and insulin production stops.

In an insulin-resistant individual, however, blood sugar does not readily enter the cells that need it, leaving blood sugar levels high. High blood sugar levels cause the pancreas to continue producing insulin in the futile attempt to satisfy the cells' needs and keep the blood sugar levels controlled. If this cycle continues long enough, there's a high probability of developing adult-onset, or type-2 diabetes.

Insulin-resistant individuals may find that their appetites aren't easily satisfied, especially at night. As they continue to eat refined products, their resistance grows worse. This causes them to store more fat while still remaining hungry (one of insulin's jobs is to make sure excess blood sugar goes *somewhere*). So it's not just a lack of willpower that drives insulin-resistant people to eat, but a physiological need expressed by cells crying out for fuel but being unable to get it even though it's "just outside." It's *real* hunger and cravings that insulin-resistant people feel. It's a *real* depletion of energy. These cravings are not imaginary! And it's not about lack of discipline or emotional hunger (although emotional hunger is also a reality for some people).

Insulin-resistant individuals should *eliminate all refined, processed carbohydrates from their diets*. This includes all non-whole carbohydrates such as bakery foods, cereals, pasta, and most grain products. Consuming whole grains means that the label does not read "enriched," "fortified," or "bleached" flour, as those terms indicate processing and you're really getting white flour. However, keep in mind that Dr. John Mercola advises insulin-resistant people to eliminate *all* grains and sugars until they regain a balance in their energy metabolism. This is because many of those with insulin resistance can't even handle "good" carbs from the pool of whole-grains. They must avoid *all* grains and sugars for a time to get back into metabolic balance.

Removing all grains and sugars from the diet until a metabolic balance reappears can be a tough regimen for those who have been over-indulging in processed carbs for years. Or perhaps all their lives. But insulin-resistant people are riding the Conveyor Belt to a Living Hell that I described in Chapter 1. *Those who want healing must do what it takes to heal.* For most people, it's not too late, but there is no magic wand. There is no magic pill that will restore the health you have lost. You will need to make lifestyle changes.

The average American consumes 170 lbs. of sugar each year. This equals 850 calories per day from sugar. Sugar consumption can boost triglyceride levels, platelet aggregation, blood pressure, and total

148

cholesterol. Sugar is one of the leading causes of heart disease in the U.S.

Q: I've heard that fruit is a simple sugar. Does this mean I should avoid all fruit?

A: Fructose is a carbohydrate found in fruit and some vegetables. And yes, it is a simple sugar. However, this type of sugar can actually enter the body's cells without depending on transportation by insulin. Therefore, it is less taxing on the pancreas (but do re-read the information about fructose dangers on page 113). Whole fruit also provides enough fiber to help avoid heavy blood sugar spikes. This means you should consume fruit in its whole state to get the complete benefit of its nutrients and fiber. Fruit juices should be cut to a minimum if not eliminated altogether since they are extremely high in calories and tend to spike blood sugar levels.

Q: If carbohydrates are such an essential part of our body's needs, why are they getting such bad press?

A: This is a phenomenon commonly referred to as "Jumping on the Band Wagon." Most authors pushing for a heavy reduction of carbohydrates apparently have little knowledge of nutrition or the necessary role that good carbohydrates play in our metabolism.

As mentioned earlier, carbohydrates help maintain a constant blood sugar level, which is essential if fat is to be burned. When you don't keep your blood sugar at a suitable level, your body goes into a survival state because its cells are sending starvation messages. Your body protects itself by pulling glycogen (stored sugar) from the liver and muscles to supply needed fuel. At the same time, it slows your metabolic rate. This leads to storing more fuel in the form of fat. Yet, if you eat the wrong types of carbohydrates in the wrong combinations with other foods, you are not able to maintain that nice, steady blood sugar level. Instead, you get spikes and valleys that are hard on the liver and pancreas. Further, the spikes and valleys drive your hormones, especially your leptin metabolism, crazy and make it impossible to maintain a lean, healthy body.

Q: My weight has dropped 15 lbs. over the last 4 weeks, but I'm still not losing the excess fat around my stomach. My personal trainer advised me to cut my calories back even further than I have been, to about 1800 calories per day. Yet, I'm still soft in the middle. Why?

A: By telling you to cut your calories, your trainer is making a grave mistake—at your expense. You're already losing more weight per week than you should be losing, which means you're losing hard-earned muscle along with other lean tissue such at bone. By cutting your calories too much, you've put your body in the *protective* mode, forcing it to use muscle for fuel. Although you've lost some pounds, *you have simultaneously slowed your metabolism.*

My advice would be to *up* your calories with whole foods in the ratios talked about on page 140. Be sure to consume those calories across your three meals (or four meals if you can't do three yet). If your trainer also has you doing more than 30 minutes of cardiovascular training at a time, you need to cut back on this. Excess cardio is not only ineffective in changing your physique (shaping your body) but can also hamper muscle growth.

Q: I've heard that digestion actually requires energy and therefore consumes calories. Do fats, carbohydrates, and proteins require the same amounts of calories to be digested?

A: Great question! And you're right. Eating the right kinds of foods helps burn calories simply by stoking the digestive process that is used to break down nutrients. Understanding this gives you even more incentive to make sure you don't short yourself on protein and carbohydrates.

Here are the figures: fat requires 5 calories per 100 consumed to digest it, carbohydrates 12 calories per 100, and protein a whopping 30 calories per 100. As you can see, dietary fats take precious little energy to digest. Further, fat carries 2.25 times more calories per gram than protein and carbohydrates. This means that, for the same number of calories, you can eat more than twice as much food in the form of protein and carbohydrates than in the form of fat. So much for the "Atkins diet," which is an abomination with respect to getting too much *saturated* fat. Yet, for metabolic reasons, fat satiates the appetite more effectively than carbs or protein. So, for any particular meal, if you have a choice about what goes into your mouth first, it should be the meal items that are heavier in fat calories.

Q: I am not a vegetarian, but I don't like to consume many meat products. I've heard you cite that animal proteins are superior. So how do I keep my protein intake up if I don't like to eat too many animal proteins?

A: Animal proteins *are* indeed superior in their protein efficiency levels—usability by the body *as protein* (as opposed to fuel for energy). Plants, however, can provide us with ample protein when combined effectively. Learning to combine plant proteins effectively may take some time and effort, but it's well worth the effort—especially for diabetics. Although animal proteins are superior in amino acid efficiency, they're also higher in the amino acid methionine. Although an essential amino acid, too much methionine can be harmful. The body converts this to a chemical called homocystein. Several good studies have linked homocystein to coronary artery disease and osteoporosis. I'm not suggesting that you avoid all animal proteins, only that you try to eat plenty of vegetables to make up for some of your daily protein percentage.

I've also talked about supplying a percentage of your protein requirements with supplemental powders. You'll find great choices on the market that include whey, casein, and egg. I personally prefer mixing casein or whey with egg to provide my body with both quick- and slow-release amino acids.

Q: What is the difference between saturated and unsaturated fats, and which are best for us?

A: The difference is saturated fats are typically more stable and solid at room temperature; and they don't react to oxidation as readily as unsaturated. Saturated fats come mostly from animals, but coconut oil is also a saturated fat. You should generally avoid *too* many saturated fats except for palm and coconut oil. Without getting too deep technically, coconut oil contains the fatty acid called lauric acid. This converts to monolaurin, the same chemical found in breast milk that protects infants. Several studies have found that coconut oil can help protect against cancer and cardiovascular disease. Coconut oil used to be declared a no-no because of its saturation status. No longer.

Unsaturated fats or oils can be subdivided into the omega-6 fatty acid (linoleic acid), found mostly in safflower and corn oil, and the omega-3 (alpha-linoleic acid), found mostly in vegetables, nuts, fish, krill, and

151

flaxseed oil. Although these fats are good for us, they should be consumed mostly in the form of whole foods and salad dressings. Processing these oils damages them and allows them to oxidize easily. Cooking further denatures oils (except coconut and palm oils), leading to damaging "free radicals" circulating throughout our bodies.

If you suffer from an inflammatory condition that you know about, try to minimize your intake of omega-6-heavy fats, as they lead to the formation of inflammatory hormone substances called eicosanoids. Omega-3 oils also lead to the formation of eicosanoids, *but of the anti-inflammatory type*. Flaxseed, fish, or krill oils are excellent choices. There's growing evidence that the extraordinarily high ratio of omega-6 to omega-3 fats in American diets is responsible for a whole lot more than inflammation: skin cancer, for example.

Q: My husband was told that his cholesterol level is borderline. Is he at risk of developing heart disease?

A: Without a complete exam and proper blood work, I can't make a clear assessment of your husband's cardiovascular health. I do think the issue of cholesterol needs clarification, however. Cholesterol isn't the main factor that increases cardiovascular risk. Did you know that nearly half of all heart attack victims have normal cholesterol values? Factors such as free radicals and inflammatory processes are what lead to the ultimate plaquing and blocking of our coronary vessels. Lipid profiles, in and of themselves, provide the physician with limited information about cardiovascular health. There are other tests that provide more pertinent information. Without getting too involved, these tests include homocysteine, lipoprotein, C-reactive protein, apolipoprotein A & B, and fibrinogen.

Q: You've included a calculation chart in your book to figure the estimated number of total calories one should consume each day. Will I always need to count my calories if I am to control my weight?

A: The calculation chart for daily calorie consumption has been included in my program to help define a base level of calorie requirements. As you begin your 12-week *Reclaim 24* Action Plan, you need to know the number of calories you're consuming each day, along with the percentages of carbs, protein, and fat. By following the guidelines and using the calculations, you are able to adjust for your individual needs. Remember, this chart provides you with specific knowledge about where you need to be. To get there, you may need to increase or decrease the number of calories defined in the guidelines due to individual factors such as genetics, changes in activity level, percentage of body fat, and hormone levels or balances.

Once you know where you stand relative to where you need to be, you'll typically follow an eating pattern that includes many of the same foods on a daily basis. While this is going on, you will have no need to count daily calories since you'll know you're working in the ballpark.

It may be better to use "look and feel" to adjust your calories from time to time. If you feel a little flat or soft, but your weight is down, you probably need to increase your calories slightly. This flat feeling is usually due to a lack of carbohydrates, which help to pull fluid into your muscles. If weight is coming off too slowly, decrease your calories by 10-15% and watch for a change. The change won't always be in the form of weight loss, but may be an increase in muscle tone or size and diminished body fat.

As mentioned earlier, because muscle is more dense than fat, you may decrease your overall size dramatically. In the meantime, your weight may drop much more moderately—and sometimes only slightly. Muscle also requires more calories to maintain than fat. So as you progress through your 12-week program, you may find that you're able to consume more calories than suggested in the calculation chart.

Q: I am very excited about beginning your 12-week program. I feel that I have the discipline to complete this, especially knowing how little time it takes from my week. What I am afraid of is that I might not have the discipline to reach and maintain my new physique.

A: You're certainly not alone. You fully understand that you must make commitments both in time and in eating habits to make this metamorphosis a permanent reality. Over a period of just a few weeks, you will learn that these new habits are not only simple to follow, but the pleasure of renewed health will strengthen them.

Statistics show that the toughest habit to change when beginning any diet and exercise program isn't the level and type of exercise, but the diet. Yes, diet is what 53% of women and 44% of men give up on after only three short weeks. This isn't necessarily a lack of discipline. Rather, it's the result of following the wrong diet. No one has the discipline to continue on a diet that ultimately leads to health issues. Our bodies are smarter than that and will readjust itself (homeostasis) when we are not getting the proper nutrients. Unfortunately, this adjustment usually entails the desire to ingest additional calories because the body tries to find sufficient nutrients in the food we eat. In other words, when the fuel is degraded, it takes more fuel to do the same job.

As long as the nutrient content of our diet is lacking, we may easily continue to crave additional food and eventually eat our way back to our beginning weight (or greater). If you're on the Atkins diet *and you have the type of metabolism that needs more carbohydrates,* most people eventually just break down and scarf up a load of carbohydrates because carbs are in short supply in the Atkins diet. Any diet that is difficult to follow regularly is probably not a great diet plan (and the Atkins plan is far from great). The same is true if a plan is terribly boring or doesn't allow for cheat days.

The lifestyle diet outlined in my program allows you to eat all the major food groups. Moreover, you're not going to be continuously hungry on this diet, always thinking about food. Over time, your body rebalances, leaving you with feelings of well-being and greater energy.

It's likely, however, that you will have *genuine* hunger for a little while before your next meal, but this is a *good* thing—especially at breakfast. It is telling you that your leptin metabolism is getting a chance to work properly and that you've been burning fat. Relish that feeling! So few people in this country are able to do so anymore.

Real hunger is not the same as the metabolic cravings that stem from leptin and insulin resistance. It's metabolic underpinnings are quite different. In fact, on the *Reclaim 24* eating plan, you learn how to distinguish genuine hunger from such cravings. One hint is that with real hunger you don't experience a large drop in your energy levels. Further, the old pleasures of frequent mouthfuls of cookies, cakes, and fast food grow less pleasurable as the body becomes more sensitive to the negative effects of processed foods and snacking. That is not to say you can't splurge a little once in a while. It just means you probably won't have the old desire to do it all the time. If you so choose, my diet plan allows you to enjoy splurge foods every fourth or fifth day. What more could you ask for this side of gluttony?

Nonetheless, it's not a good idea to allow real hunger to run for more than 30 to 45 minutes before taking your next meal. If you do, a metabolic shift occurs that tells your brain starvation may be happening.

After a few such episodes, your body enters "energy conservation mode." Your metabolism slows down, your fat stores begin to increase, and your energy level drops. This is what happens to people who habitually skip meals. So you learn how to eat enough quality food during each meal to get you almost all the way through to the next meal—but not more!

Q: What happens if I make little or no progress after 12 weeks with your *Reclaim 24* Action Plan? I've been devoted to other diet and fitness programs in the past but have failed with all of them even though I've followed their approaches to the tee. I'm at the end of my rope!

A: There is genuine hope if you think you're at the end of your rope! I'm answer your question at great length in the next chapter.

Stress Damage: It actually starts building when you are in your teens and early twenties, but you don't notice it so much, if at all. Yet it keeps on building. Then one morning when you least expect it, you look into the mirror and wonder who you're looking at ...

"Who is that imposter?"

It can ruin your day, and maybe many days to follow.

What you need to know, right now, is that you can slow down stress buildup—dramatically. And even reverse much of what has already taken place. And you need to know that even as the calendar years pass, you don't have to experience the debilitating effects of stress buildup that destroy your quality of life decades before nature intended. You *can* take another pathway if you don't like what you see happening to yourself or those around you!

13: But What if It's Not Working?

If you, *either a man or woman,* have been an honest and diligent practitioner of the *Reclaim 24* Action Plan and have found little or no success with weight loss or change in appearance, and if this isn't the first time you've experienced such disappointment after working so hard, then be cautious. The all-too-human truth is this:

> **Most people in your shoes continue to react in ways that more often than not result in greater weight gain and emotional devastation! Why is that? Because <u>the emotional distress that comes with body distortion and premature aging</u> *begs* <u>for relief—NOW</u>! What's more, the desire for quick relief simply overwhelms rational thinking about possible long-term damage and failure.**

You are a most likely a candidate for the help of a qualified wellness professional and health mentor!

Let's face it: for many overweight people, this is a desperate struggle. For such desperation, anything that seems to offer a quick, easy answer to weight loss or other health and fitness problems is a straw worth grasping for. But that's precisely the problem. Everywhere you look, people are offering you only straws to grasp, straws that come with great promises of quick, easy solutions (but their legal disclaimers about "atypical" results ultimately tell the truth). Somehow, the promises just don't pan out because straws—no matter what shiny, new, expensive packages they come wrapped in—are still straws!

And now about *your* efforts. How are you feeling about yourself when you see little or no change despite working so hard? Are you tired and discouraged with the continued struggle and loss of vitality? <u>Are you thoroughly disappointed yet</u>? Enough, already …

You need to re-educate yourself with the *shocking scientific facts that have emerged in the last few years*. The missing link to a more youthful appearance—to radically increased levels of energy and a greater quality of life—is now within your grasp. But you must understand how fat is burned and health is created. There's no simple way around this if you have a stubborn weight problem. You must understand the latest facts that science has revealed, facts that prove what we've known all along: some folks, no matter how hard they work out, how healthfully they feed themselves, or how much they starve themselves, <u>cannot lose fat</u>! The key to solving this heartbreak is to do what it takes to understand how <u>your</u> type of metabolism can be forced into burning off unwanted fat and cellulite. And unless you're a "rugged individual," you will seek a professional who can help you achieve your weight-loss goal, healthfully, using a fact-based program. You already know about much of the health side from digging into my *Reclaim 24* Action Plan. This helps you *permanently* succeed in your efforts with much less stress and strain on your physical and emotional well-being.

To get you up-to-speed, let's first start with the most common weight-loss myths, plus the facts you need to know to dispel those myths.

You Must Be Able to Distinguish Myth from Fact

MYTH: Overweight is a disease that leads to other diseases.

FACT: Overweight is a <u>symptom</u> of diminished wellness, the same diminished wellness that eventually leads to common diseases such as hardened or clogged arteries, hypertension, stroke, and diabetes. Yes, certain types of body fat (especially belly fat) are more dangerous than others because of metabolic over-signaling by the hormone leptin; yet we must regard fat or obesity as a *secondary* cause of disease. The first cause is the set of conditions that creates the excess fat stores in the first place.

If you're smart, you'll recognize that being overweight is a symptom of things going wrong in your body. You'll recognize that the urges you have to "misbehave" with poor diet are really powerful biological urges whose days will be numbered if you get yourself into a <u>fact-based</u> program tailored to your individual needs!

MYTH: The main purpose of body fat is to insulate and cushion you.

FACT: Fat is a form of energy that the body stores because chemical messages are telling it to. In overweight people who can't lose fat, those messages are getting screwed up.

MYTH: Eating fat makes you fat.

FACT: No. It's the inability to burn fat that makes you fat. Chronically overweight people tend to burn carbs, but they burn stored fat only with great difficulty, *IF AT ALL*. That's right, some people's hormones are *so* far out of whack that they can store fat but not retrieve and burn it! You see them in the news. It takes the right knowledge and a measured effort to become a <u>fat burner</u>. It doesn't happen by itself.

MYTH: To lose weight, just cut calories.

FACT: Cutting calories is the answer to weight loss *only if you're already in good health and have a diet and exercise program tailored to your physical makeup and stress levels.* For most people with stubborn weight, the <u>very last thing</u> they should be doing is cutting calories because it doesn't work. IT DOESN'T WORK! By the way, did I say IT DOESN'T WORK?

MYTH: But many people are losing weight on modern weight-loss diets, aren't they?

FACT: At the University of California, the world's largest study of weight loss has shown that *diets do not work for the vast majority of dieters and may even put lives at risk.* "You can initially lose 5 to 10 per cent of your weight on any number of diets," says researcher Dr. Traci Mann, "But after this honeymoon period, the weight comes back. We found that the majority of people regained all the weight, plus more. Sustained weight loss was found only in a small minority of participants, while complete weight regain was found in the majority."

The UC researchers analyzed the results of more than 30 studies involving thousands of dieters. Although the overview did not name specific weight-loss plans, some of the more popular diets in recent years have included the low-carbohydrate, high-protein Atkins diet, South Beach, LA Weight Loss, Nutrisystems, Weight Watchers, Slim-Fast, Mediterranean, and the GI diet (which is rich in wholegrain carbohydrates). Some of the specific findings:

❑ While most lose some pounds initially, more than two-thirds pile the pounds straight back on—and quickly. They end up heavier than they did at the start. <u>It's the vicious cycle of going from fat to fatter</u>—losing the same weight over and over again, and then gaining back even more! Further, the extra stress placed on the body by repeated weight loss and gain means most people are better off not dieting at all.

❑ Dr. Mann's research showed that up to two-thirds of dieters put on all the weight they lost—and more—in the following four to five years. Half of those taking part in one study were more than 11 lbs. heavier five years later, while dieters taking part in another study actually *ended up heavier than other volunteers who hadn't tried to lose weight.*

❑ Research has shown that repeated, rapid weight gain and loss associated with dieting can double the risk of death from heart disease—including heart attacks—and the risk of premature death in general. Such yo-yo weight loss has also been linked to stroke and diabetes and shown to suppress the immune system, making the body more vulnerable to infection.

MYTH: If you can't lose weight and keep it off, there's something wrong with your willpower and discipline.

FACT: If you can't lose weight and keep it off, it's because there's something wrong with your health! Millions of people in this country experience strong and continually distracting hunger urges even though they are taking in more than the number of calories they need to sustain their body weight. These are powerful biological urges that stem from hormonal imbalances. Most will tell you that it's as if they have a

> **It's almost impossible to eat less when there's a little devil on your shoulder, born from a hormonal imbalance, that's constantly whispering to you, 'eat more, get fatter.'**

little devil on their shoulder constantly whispering: "Eat more, get fatter." (That's your imbalanced leptin metabolism speaking.) There's only one solution: You must get that devil off your shoulder!

When you follow a scientific, fact-based program, you are able to balance your hormones and get your glands, diet, and exercise levels into the health zone. Your cravings then moderate for greater fitness, appearance, and overall health.

MYTH: The *real* secret to weight loss is moderation in all things.

FACT: False, false, false. If you have a stubborn weight problem, moderation won't work for you until you get healthy. In fact, moderation may be impossible while that hormone devil is whispering in your ear. Further, when it comes to weight-loss programs, *one size does not fit all,* despite what all the fads and authorities have told you. Different body types and different hormone-rebalancing challenges need different solutions. You *must* tailor your approach to you, and you *must* know how to tailor it!

Do you know what weight-loss solution is best for your body type? Do you even know what your body type is and why your extra weight hangs on you the way it does? Believe it or not, how your extra weight distributes itself on you tells us which glands and hormones are creating your stubborn weight-loss problems and what you must do to reverse the downward spiral (and the extra downward pressure on the floor).

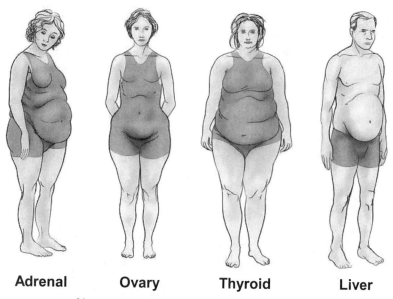

Adrenal   Ovary   Thyroid   Liver

Take a look.[26] Do you see your body shape in the above picture? Are you tired of belly fat? Bulges? Lumps? Exercise with little if any reward? (By the way, each of the shown body types can be found in either men or women. For men, the "ovary" type means estrogen dominance.)

MYTH: Exercising along with eating healthful foods is the key to permanent weight loss.

FACT: Getting closer to the truth. But if you don't get the *right type* of exercise and healthy foods for your body type and metabolism, your form of exercise and food choices can actually <u>prevent</u> you from losing weight, or even make you gain it. You <u>must</u> know what type of exercise and foods are right for YOU. Further, you need to go beyond just diet and exercise for lifelong success.

---

[26] Permission granted to use body type images by Dr. Eric Berg, author of *The 7 Principles of Fat Burning* (Action Publishing, 2006) p. 7.

The Four Essentials for Achieving <u>Permanent</u> Weight Loss

- **Body-Type Assessment**
- **Hormone Assessment**
- **Stress Management**
- **Health Rebuilding**

Hormones control your metabolism. You need to know how to rally your hormones to work in your favor instead of against you, and you need to know how to do that in a long-term, health-building way. Most important, you need to know what makes your metabolism stubborn to deal with. If you find yourself in a chronic overweight condition despite past diets, it's because your own hormones have been working against you, making you fat and distorting your body's shape. You need to find out which hormones and glands are determining your body appearance before you can effectively make the changes you long for.

You have six fat-burning and three fat-storing hormones. Further, some of those fat-burning hormones also have an anti-aging effect that we all welcome with open arms.

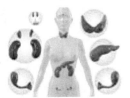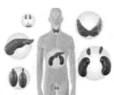

Different things trigger each hormone. Do you know what those triggers are? Do you know where you stand? You want to be able to trigger all six fat-burning hormones for best effect, and send the fat-storing hormones on vacation. So how do you do that?

Here's a hint; it's going to involve the foods you eat, the type of exercise you do, and the kinds of stress you put yourself under. Further, it's going to involve breaking more old habits *that you may not even know you have*. Chapters 4 and 5 will continue to help you with that.

Just remember, <u>stubborn weight such as belly fat isn't the primary problem</u>! It's just a symptom that your glands are not healthy and your hormones are unbalanced. Further, excess fat isn't a disease in and of itself. Rather, it's a symptom of diminished wellness. <u>You must correct the right problem for long-term success</u>. Sadly, many overweight people try to lose this unwanted, embarrassing fat by starving themselves, taking

162

an excessive number of pills, or both. Such shortcuts have been proven time and again to be next to worthless. Yet, overweight people often see themselves as healthy exceptions, with stubborn weight being their only problem (and many will stick to this story compulsively). In truth, there's likely to be no real help for them in their permanent weight-loss mission. You see, they are not healthy, they are unwilling to consider the possibility that they are not healthy, and they are unwilling to make the effort to become healthy. That's a tough combination to work with. Don't be such a person.

Dr. Eric Berg relates the problem of a 400-pound woman who had driven from Michigan to his clinic in Virginia for a consultation to help her lose weight.[27] He found out she was having only one bowel movement a month (yikes!), which meant her liver function was quite poor. He explained that her bowels had to start working better before she could lose weight. He never saw her again. Her bowel problem wasn't a concern of hers. She was more interested in weight loss. Do you see how a compulsion can overwhelm rational thinking?

The emotions tied up in being overweight can be terribly strong. But the truth is you have to do many wrong things to get to 400 pounds, and you have to do them for a long, long time. Now all she wanted to do was treat the fat symptom while her organs were failing at their jobs and speeding her demise. She probably went for gastric bypass surgery. It's not surprising that so many people die following that procedure. Excess fat may be the least of their problems, and the surgery just turns out to be the extra stress that breaks the camel's back.

So, to do it right, you need to light upon the right diet and exercise program for your body type, and this includes learning how to use food and activity to trigger all your fat-burning hormones while suppressing your fat-storing hormones. You need to locate your stressors and decide what to do about them. And finally, you need to rally your subconscious mind to help you out in the most practical of situations. A tall order, to be sure, but within your grasp.

Will You Be Able to Work This All Out for Yourself?

Well, maybe—if you have a research temperament and you're in no special hurry to start turning your life around. But it sure can be daunting

---

[27] Eric Berg, DC, *The 7 Principles of Fat Burning* (Los Angeles, Action Publishing, 2006) 99.

to successfully manage weight and appearance while also improving fitness, energy, mood, and longevity. Hundreds of approaches, programs, systems, and fads are touted to help us develop health and fitness. So, how do you sort all this out while still retaining your sanity? How do you tell the difference between myth, fad, and solid advice? How do you know what fits *you* best?

As I suggested at the beginning of this chapter, please seek out a professional wellness mentor who can take you—someone with a stubborn weight problem—one step beyond the *Reclaim 24* Action Plan to a specialized area tailored for you. Someone who can show you the most direct path to your goal with the least amount of wear and tear on your being. But caution is in order; there could be a problem here.

Rare, indeed, are mentors <u>fully</u> qualified to help others achieve *permanent* weight loss in *healthy ways*. Sure, you can find plenty of weight loss "coaches" around to help you stay on track with certain diet plans, but as you know by now, diets, drugs, and surgery only work in the short term—and only sometimes. They almost *never* build lifelong health.

I truly wish I could give you even better advice than this from afar, but that's not the purpose of *Metamorphosis*. This book, especially this chapter and the information in Part III, already gives you a tremendous advantage over others with stubborn weight problems. Not that you want or need an advantage over others. But it does means you've made a considerable effort to get yourself to this point and, for someone in your boat, you now see the many of the pitfalls out there and how to avoid them. I can only have great admiration for you.

As things stand, this book has given you plenty of justification for holding a lifelong passion for wellness so you can **rewrite your life experience** (and perhaps the life experiences of your family members and others you love). Knowing what I do about life, I'm sure that if you continue to hold that passion for wellness and do the common-sense things that you read about here, life will miraculously show you the way. "Follow your nose," as they say. That's how it works.

Having said that, I want you to have *plenty* of understanding about hormones and wellness before you seek a professional mentor or wellness doctor. In this way, you will be able to make better choices. I've written Chapter 14 to help you with such choices.

14: The Role of Hormones in Wellness
(Definitely Not Just for Women!)

"The overall deterioration of the body that comes with growing old is not inevitable... We now realize that some aspects of it can be prevented or reversed."[28]

You probably know this by now, but I'll repeat it for emphasis: Stress is one of the main causes of hormone imbalance and slow metabolism in our society. Although a certain level of stress is normal and even essential for both mental and physical development, too much "distress" causes an overload syndrome that leads to the deterioration of your health and rapid "aging."

In many ways, we have more stress today than ever before. Modern developments such as e-mail, cell phones, laptop computers, genetically engineered food, "super-sized" food portions, junk food, caffeine, and the lack of physical activity increase our overall stress load. People are working longer and harder with little to show for it. Over 60% of Americans take no annual vacation. Physical education programs have been drastically reduced or eliminated in some of our schools. For those schools that continue to offer P.E., students often have the choice not to participate.

Kids are no longer playing outside. They have instead chosen to stay indoors and occupy their minds by watching television (idiot box), playing video games, or parking their rear ends in front of the computer for hours on end chatting with friends or surfing the Internet. The result of all these "advances" has led to a society that is fatter and sicker than ever before. More and more stress, fewer and fewer health-building remedies.

The pressures of stress can come from mental (emotional), chemical, and physical sources. Interestingly, the body has the same biochemical response to different types of stress. For example, if you're stuck in traffic and stressed about being late for work, the biochemical response is identical to the response activated by lack of sleep, too much physical work, or an allergic reaction to food. Our bodies were never designed for

---

[28] Daniel Rudman, M.D. *New England Journal of Medicine*, Volume 323 July 5, 1990 Number 1

repeated, chronic bouts of stress, day in and day out. We were designed to run away from the tiger and then relax and recuperate. But recuperation isn't happening in society today. Increased workloads, too little rest, too many deadlines, processed foods, and chemicals in our environment all lead to the cumulative effect and the "stress response."

Physiologically, when we are stressed out, our adrenal glands release greater-than-normal amounts of a hormone called cortisol. Stressors can include extremely low-calorie diets, intense physical training, high-volume training, lack of quality sleep, job pressures, fights with your spouse, or being caught in a traffic jam. Trauma, injury, and surgery also serve as major stressors to the body.

This unique hormone, cortisol, allows our bodies to adapt to the increased energy demands of stress. But the release of cortisol from our adrenal glands is only intended to handle acute bursts of stress, not continuous flows. Prolonged and chronic stress leads to what has been termed "chronic stress syndrome." This syndrome is a condition in which your body's adrenal glands continuously release cortisol in response to ongoing stress. Initially your body is able to produce these elevated levels of cortisol, but with time the adrenals fatigue and lose their ability to keep up with the demand. Then the levels of cortisol become depressed and blood sugar levels drop, creating hunger and exhaustion.

This pattern typically occurs in individuals who frequently miss meals (especially breakfast), who eat and drink many processed carbohydrates, and who fuel themselves during the day with caffeine. They notice some degree of insomnia or don't feel rested upon awakening. Further, they get sick more often, develop chronic fatigue, experience more frequent aches and pains, and see their abdominal girth getting larger than their hip girth. They may even eat less and exercise more than they did a few years ago, but they're still unable to lose weight.

And then there's that mid-day crash. It comes around 2:30 to 3:30, making them feel like taking a nap or grabbing an espresso from Starbucks to keep them going.

Does this sound like you?

We really don't understand the full impact of how chronic stress affects our health. It's a silent killer of large proportions. Compare our society with the European. Europeans don't work the long hours we do. They typically take two or three-hour breaks in the afternoon, and most take at least a month off for vacation each year. Their food is freshly picked and does not come in boxes. Fast food has not become a staple of their diets and they spend more time walking instead of driving everywhere. If you ever have an opportunity to visit Europe, you'll notice the majority of fat or obese you see are visiting Americans! Europeans simply don't have the rates of obesity, diabetes, cardiovascular disease, or other diseases linked to stress that Americans do (except in the U.K., which is now competing very well with the U.S. in rates of obesity and declining health).

Insulin Resistance and Its Relationship to Diabetes

As you may recall from earlier chapters, I talked about "insulin resistance" and its potentially negative effects on health and body metamorphosis. So, exactly what is this condition and how do you know if you have it?

Well, first off, let's just say that this condition is more common in this country than you might have guessed. In fact, it's estimated that 25-35% of the United States population has some degree of insulin resistance. Now that's a scary figure when you realize that a large percentage of these people eventually develop type-2 diabetes, now an epidemic. What follows is a layman's explanation of how this condition develops.

Glucose is a simple blood sugar that serves as your body's main energy source. Every time you eat, your body's digestive process converts some of your food into glucose. This additional glucose enters your bloodstream. The hormone, insulin, which is made in the pancreas, is then released to transport the extra blood glucose into your cells to be used for energy creation. Remember, lean cells create more energy than fat cells, by quite a margin.

The food-to-glucose conversion process, along with the delivery of glucose to cells by insulin, works extremely well as long as your blood glucose levels don't "spike up" too often or too high. When you choose your foods carefully and consume a diet similar to that recommended in my nutrition program, your blood sugar levels jump very little and remain within a narrow range, balanced by the action of insulin. Under these conditions, the pancreas is able to secrete insulin in small spurts throughout the day. This allows the pancreas to operate within its "biologically comfortable" support zone, not placing much stress on it.

Moreover, by keeping insulin levels low, cell receptors that respond to insulin are not over-stimulated.[29] You can think of cell receptors as front-line "molecular guards" that only accept visitors with the right credentials.

However, processed carbs—so prevalent in the American diet— require little time and digestive "overhead" to be broken down into glucose and dumped into the bloodstream. Therefore, processed carbs place almost immediate demands on the pancreas to produce insulin in relatively large amounts. This happens because a healthy body inherently recognizes high levels of blood glucose to be dangerous[30] and therefore does something about it, fast. So, bursts of insulin work to get blood glucose back to normal, safer levels.

When blood glucose levels spike often, two problems emerge. The first problem is that the pancreas has to pump out insulin beyond its biological comfort zone and with time can "burn out" from being overtaxed. This can lead to diminished insulin production and eventually type-1 (insulin dependent) diabetes.

The second problem is that cell receptors eventually become desensitized to frequent, elevated bursts of insulin and therefore less effective at allowing proper amounts of glucose into the protected cells. In other words, these "molecular guards" start turning away greater numbers of credentialed "visitors" and glucose can no longer be transported into the needy cells as easily. This condition is called *insulin resistance*. It can and does lead to type-2 diabetes, formerly called non-insulin-dependent or "adult-onset" diabetes.

But glucose rejected by resistant cells doesn't just disappear. It either remains in the bloodstream, with time creating *major* problems in and of itself, or insulin carries it to fat cells where it is converted to fatty acids and stored for later use (and for all the world to see). When things get really bad, some excess glucose is dumped in the urine.

But why will fat cells accept glucose when lean, energy-burning cells won't? Because fat cells develop insulin resistance *later* than lean cells.

---

[29] The over-stimulation of a cell's receptors to *any* chemical in the body leads to a decreased sensitivity that is the hallmark of physical dependence. This usually means more and more of the same chemical is needed to get the same response from the body's cells. Caffeine dependence is an example.

[30] Long-term complications such as eye disease, kidney disease, heart attacks, strokes, and more.

This delay provides the body with a safety "cushion" because excess blood glucose can be swept away to fat stores. So, even people with mild insulin resistance will be able to store fat easily—for a limited time, anyway—to protect against high levels of blood glucose.

With type-1 diabetes, the pancreas can no longer make sufficient amounts of insulin to do its job. If untreated, it may lead to neuropathies (nerve destruction), vascular deterioration (requiring amputations), blindness, coma, and even death. Do I need to say more about these "conveyor-belt-to-living-hell" conditions? Type-1 diabetics must take insulin and should not play Russian roulette with poor diets loaded with processed carbohydrates.

On the other hand, type-2 diabetes can most often be avoided and even reversed. This is a milder form of diabetes that does not require exogenous insulin. Yet, it can lead to serious health consequences and even type-1 diabetes if not corrected. By the way, sufficient exercise is one of the best ways to reduce insulin resistance *for life*.

When insulin resistance prevents sufficient glucose from getting into the cells to produce energy, the common signs and symptoms include fatigue, mental fogginess, depression, and the inability to lose weight. Insulin-resistant people also complain of irritability when they miss meals. They crave sweets and caffeine.

If you're suffering from insulin resistance, you may have tried exercise and diet in the past but eventually became discouraged and quit because you couldn't lose weight. A typical sign of insulin resistance that correlates to high cardiovascular risk—especially in females—is a waist girth larger than hip girth.

Now, going back to cortisol, the hormone that responds to stress. It does this by inducing your cells to release fuel into your bloodstream where it can be used by other cells, especially muscle cells, that need it to handle physically stressful moments—like having to jump out of the way of a car bearing down on you. But if stress causes the release of fuel into the bloodstream and the fuel doesn't have anywhere to go, then guess what? Insulin production spikes to escort the unneeded fuel out of the bloodstream and into fat storage, just as it does when we eat a meal high in processed carbs. Thus, the overabundance of cortisol leads to both insulin resistance and fat storage.

Prolonged, elevated cortisol levels not only induce insulin resistance but also leptin resistance. Leptin is a hormone produced by white fat

169

cells. One of its functions is to tell the brain to decrease food intake. The more fat cells that are present, especially in certain parts of the body, the more leptin is produced to notify the brain that starvation isn't an issue with this particular body. This is how leptin helps to regulate fat storage. It carries the satiation message.

However, brain-cell receptors can become insensitive to leptin, just as body cells become insensitive to insulin. If this happens, the potential for obesity rises dramatically because leptin's satiation messages aren't reaching home. Hunger pangs continue even when additional calories aren't needed; extra sugar enters the bloodstream but can't be used by the cells; insulin stores the excess sugar as fat; leptin signals continue to spike to tell the brain to decrease food intake; the leptin spikes make brain-cell receptors for leptin even more insensitive; and the vicious cycle continues with hunger still present. To make matters worse, if too much stress exhausts the adrenals and cortisol levels plummet, then hypoglycemia arises, inducing even more cravings. What a mess!

So, these vicious cycles are kicked off by stress, the over-consumption of processed carbohydrates, and the lack of enough exercise to lower insulin resistance. When these factors are brought into balance so that cortisol, insulin, and leptin can function as intended, the result is a leaner, more energetic body.

The overall impact of prolonged stress on human physiology and metabolism is beyond the scope of this book. I've only touched on those factors related to body composition and weight management. Other detrimental factors include thyroid disorders, liver detoxification dysfunction, digestive disorders, suppressed immune function, decreased bone density, depression, insomnia, neurodegenerative disease, and cardiovascular disease. Bottom line: prolonged stress is perilous. We need to learn how to reduce it or handle it better. That's what a wellness lifestyle is all about.

More on Essential Fatty Acids

I mentioned the importance of essential fatty acids (EFAs) in Chapter 11 because they are required for fat metabolism. I now want to further elaborate their importance on hormone function and in handling inflammation responses.

Studies have shown that inadequate EFAs such as DHA (docoasahexaenidic acid) lead to altered cell signaling[31]. This means that hormones may be having an exaggerated or diminished response on the body even though lab results show normal hormone ranges. This is why my patients may have symptoms of hormone imbalance even though lab tests come back negative. Further, it explains why some who receive hormone replacement therapy fail to have the responses expected.

EFA metabolism disorders as well as EFA deficiencies are common in the United States. Researchers have estimated that up to 80% of the U.S. population receives inadequate daily intake of EFAs. The American diet is seriously deficient in essential fatty acids due to mass commercial refinements of fats and oil products, and the production of foods containing unnatural fats such as trans fatty acids. These substitutes for the real thing are employed because their structure makes commercial processing easier. They also possess a longer shelf life. Good for commercial interests, not so good for you.

In addition to proper intake of EFAs and the factors that alter EFA metabolism, a balance must exist between the omega-6 and omega-3 fats for optimal cellular response and function. The ideal ratio of omega-6 to omega-3 EFAs is between 3:1 and 5:1.[32] Some researchers even believe the ideal ratio is lower, and any value above 4:1 leads to health problems. Yet, in the U.S., the ratios have commonly been reported as high as 25:1. Some higher.

Here's an important point. The overabundance of commonly available omega-6 acids contributes to a low-grade inflammatory process in the body. We see this clinically in conditions such as fibromyalgia, lupus, and other chronic pain syndromes. Even skin cancer appears to be promoted by an overabundance of omega-6 EFAs.[33]

One more thing. A high level of omega-6 reduces the body's ability to use omega 3s. Omega 3s promote fat-burning while also inhibiting the calories that we do consume from being stored as fat. There's certainly something to be said for that!

---

[31] Mandaell, A.J., "Non-equilibrium Behavior of Some Brain Enzyme Receptor Systems." *Annu Rev Pharmacol Toxicol* 1984;24;237-274

[32] Shamberger, R.J., "Erythrocyte Fatty Acid Studies in Patients.", J Advance Med 1997;10(3):195-205

[33] *Proceedings of the National Academy of Sciences*, June 19, 2001, vol. 98, no. 13: 7510-7515

Both Women and Men Can Improve Hormone Function!

In the late 1980's, Stephen De Felice, M.D., coined the term *neutriceutical* to describe chemicals in foods that have medicinal power. These include vitamins, minerals, amino acids, herbs, and semi-vitamins. Neutriceutical formulas have also been shown to help counter inflammation, optimize gene expression, prevent damage to genes, and repair DNA after damage has already been done. Fortunately, some neutriceuticals are designed to stimulate the production of certain hormones in order to achieve an eventual, natural systemic balance (homeostasis). That's why I employ neutriceuticals in my practice.

Before prescribing any designed neutriceutical or formula to any of my patients, I have them first complete a "Metabolic Assessment Form." This is a thorough and precise questionnaire designed to allow me to identify, among other things, failing hormonal systems. This assessment helps to eliminate unnecessary testing while more accurately identifying the obvious deficiencies that a patient may be experiencing. It helps me "zero in" to likely areas of distress.

Following this, further hormonal tests can validate the initial assessment findings and provide information to design the best hormonal rebalancing approach for the patient's situation. The majority of hormonal tests can be completed in the privacy of a patient's home and don't require blood draws. No dreaded trips to the phlebotomist to get stuck! More on this in a few pages.

Female Hormone Changes

Well, there's just no getting around it—sex hormones decline with time, for both men and women. And with females, this can certainly throw a ratchet in the whole weight management thing. If you're over 40 and finding it ever more difficult to keep your desired figure, you may be entering the beginning stages of menopause. If you're still in your younger years, pay attention! You too will soon need to face these upcoming changes. It's better to be educated and prepared than to suffer unrelenting anxiety from the unknown.

So what exactly is menopause? As a woman approaches middle age, the ovaries begin to lose their ability to produce the sex hormones estrogen and progesterone. As these hormones decline, physiological changes begin to take place indicating that the childbearing years are nearing an end. Some of the most common changes include loss of

172

sexual desire, weight gain, vaginal dryness, loss of breast tissue (and thus fullness), dry skin, insomnia, depression, and irritability. Of course, menstruation ceases. Every woman is affected differently. For some it can be quite devastating. For others, it's just a part of life and a minor obstacle to push through and adapt to. Either way, it's a condition that definitely impedes, at some level, the progress of body metamorphosis.

Does this mean you are fighting a losing battle? Absolutely not! It does mean, however, that the road may be a bit bumpier and a little longer. But with persistence, discipline, and smart choices, you can still attain your goal.

So, what are some of these choices? First, follow the program outlined in this book. It's been carefully designed. Your falling sex hormone levels play only a minor role in managing your health and figure as compared to the other factors discussed so far. Nevertheless, the falling levels do have an impact. The good thing is that you can help resolve this problem naturally, without resorting to synthetic hormone replacement.

Bio-Identical Hormones

Up until recently, hormone replacement was predominately achieved through the use of synthetics derived from plants and then altered. Now things have changed. Have you heard of the pharmaceutical Premarin®? The name for this product was derived from its chemical foundation: pregnant mare urine. Doesn't that strike you as odd? I don't know about you, but I think there should be better, more natural, human-oriented methods for designing and replacing human hormones than starting with the urine of pregnant mares.

Well guess what? There are such methods! In fact, hormones chemically identical to those found in humans can also be found other places in nature. So why are the pharmaceutical giants not preparing and promoting them? Why are they modifying pregnant mare urine for consumption by women instead of providing hormones that the body is designed to use?

Because they can't patent products that already occur in nature.

This means they'd have to compete with dozens of other manufacturers able to deliver the same products plucked from nature's bounty. There would be no huge profit that normally comes from being the sole provider of a patented chemical.

173

Pharmaceutical companies make their money by designing synthetic, unique products, thereby earning patents that keep the competition out of the game for quite a few years. The problem is that these synthetics don't match the body's own hormones. The result is they create health problems because the body doesn't know how to handle them.

The next thing you know you're taking another patent drug to try to counteract the health problems created by the first one. And this cycle can certainly repeat—and does with alarming frequency. Some people have their dresser tops or kitchen counters strewn with drugstore containers. Our poor bodies!

In contrast to products like Premarin, *real* estrogen and progesterone do not suddenly become harmful to a woman in her 50's when, in her earlier years, those same hormones were mandatory for normal health, sex characteristics, well-being, and general function. It's the altered forms of hormones that create the mayhem and damage of side effects. This is because the altered forms, in addition to doing what's intended by chemists, fool cell receptors (you know, the "molecular guards") into accepting other types of unintended influences that can do damage. It's like welcoming marauders at the front door because they are disguised as friends.

Thankfully there are more and more pharmacists working to provide hormones in their naturally occurring state. These individuals are called "compounding pharmacists." That description more closely identifies with what pharmacists were originally intended to be. Compounding pharmacists are well-educated professionals who have a thorough understanding of body chemistry and physiology. They typically work with a group of physicians who are also well-versed in more natural approaches to hormone replacement.

Beware any physician who prescribes hormones, whether synthetic or bio-identical, who doesn't test you beforehand to determine your present levels. This is madness—no more than a guessing game based on subjective symptoms that can go from one extreme to the other. Victims of such poor physician practice eventually become frustrated and simply choose to abandon their efforts altogether, accepting their state of being.

The bottom line is this: if you wish to further evaluate bio-identical replacement, seek out a doctor who understands blood, saliva, and urine testing. When it comes to properly evaluating your hormone levels, saliva testing is quickly becoming the front-runner.

Laboratory Methods and Testing

We have three different mediums for testing hormones. They are saliva, serum, and urine. Each test has its advantages and disadvantages. When I use saliva testing, my patients collect their samples in the privacy of their own homes and send them directly to the lab for processing.

Saliva tests appear to be the most popular of the three tests in recent years. They are better than serum tests for three reasons.

First, they are less expensive because they don't require the services of blood-draw specialists such as phlebotomists or nurses. And of course, you don't have to waste time or fuel traveling to a facility and waiting in line to "get stuck."

Second, one saliva test will get you the information that two serum tests require. Serum tests require extra lab procedures to filter out the protein-bound hormones before the bioavailable fraction can be measured accurately. At their simplest, serum tests are usually measurements of hormones bound to carrier proteins such as sex-hormone-binding globulin, albumin, thyroid-binding hormone, and so on. Therefore, they don't give direct information about the relative quantity of *active* hormones available to receptors. Rather, *those values are estimated*—not such a good idea in many cases because estimates can be far enough off the mark to create problems. Of course, additional serum tests are available to measure the free-hormone fractions, but the tests are costly.

In contrast, saliva tests "filter out" protein-bound hormones right up front. They measure only bioavailable, non-protein-bound hormones—the free-fractioned portions that are actually available for your tissues to use. *This is the knowledge that clinicians need.* It tells them how much of a hormone is actually left for binding to the hormone receptors of cells. After all, that's how hormones induce a physiological response. Protein-bound hormones on the other hand are inert—already used up, so to speak. Knowing their levels doesn't help a clinician very much.

Third, saliva tests can be used to measure daily rhythms of hormones such as cortisol; also hormone changes over an entire menstrual cycle. Such tests require continuous sampling that would be inconvenient, at best, if you had to visit a lab to draw every sample—morning, noon, afternoon, and night (for cortisol). Doing it at home is a piece of cake—or maybe a handful of nuts.

However, saliva tests can't be used for *all* hormones, including hormone-structured compounds such as thyroid-binding globulin. Sadly, even when they can be used, outdated healthcare services generally don't understand the advantages of saliva testing or how to apply it.

Urine tests are also available to measure hormones, but what they measure needs to be understood. Urine tests basically measure hormones and hormone metabolites *after they have undergone detoxification by the liver.* Such measurements provide both advantages and disadvantages. On the negative side, urinary hormone tests are not terribly reliable for determining the amount or rate of hormones produced by organs and glands. This is because amounts detected are affected by the tested individual's detoxification and "clearance" rates—rates that can vary significantly across different people. On the positive side, the fact that urinary hormone tests reflect clearance and detoxification means they can accurately measure hormone metabolites.

Stimulating Your Own Hormone Production

Maybe you're too young for hormone replacement or you simply wish to avoid it altogether. Can you still keep your own system functioning at its best?

Absolutely!

But before reviewing options, it's important (if you're a woman—and probably also if you're a man) that you have a deep understanding of the condition called menopause. This knowledge or understanding allows you to work with your doctor to design the proper plan. You should never be in the dark when it comes to altering your hormone balance, whether stimulating production or depressing it. The practice of wellness doesn't do so well in the dark! Although the following discussion is necessarily technical in nature, do try to get a sense of how everything works together so you can see how intricate hormone balance and homeostasis are in the body. The intricacy should tell you that you don't want to be fooling with your hormones without professional support!

As I stated earlier, menopause is associated with a decline in the female sex hormones estrogen and progesterone. These hormones are produced in the ovaries, which are under the influence of follicle stimulating hormone (FSH) and leutinizing hormone (LH). FSH and LH are produced in the brain—specifically the anterior pituitary. The production of FSH and LH is under the influence of another section of the brain called the hypothalamus, which constantly monitors the total amount of estrogen and progesterone circulating in the body.

When these sex hormone levels are low, the hypothalamus directs the anterior pituitary to increase the output of either LH or FSH. This in turn has a direct effect on the ovaries in their production of estrogen or progesterone. As these hormone levels rise to their peaks, the hypothalamus instructs the anterior pituitary to shut off production of LH or FSH and the ovaries slow production. In medical terms, this is called a "negative feedback loop" and is part of homeostasis control.

This feedback system works marvelously throughout the first half of a woman's life. Then things begin to change. Most commonly, the ovaries start to lose their ability to keep up, despite the influence of FSH and LH. Eventually, even FSH and LH decline, resulting in a permanently lower production of progesterone and estrogen.

The good news is that you have a back-up system. That's right. Remember the discussion on adrenal function earlier in this chapter? Those two small glands sitting on top of your kidneys take over the ovaries' job when hormone production slows or even stops. The adrenals continue to provide small amounts of progesterone, estrogen, and even testosterone well into your later years (they produce small amounts even in a woman's younger years). Although the adrenals help out, they don't have the ability to produce these hormones at the pre-menopausal levels. Nor are they under the influence of FSH and LH.

* * *

Congratulations! You now have a more thorough understanding of female hormone function than just about anyone, *even many doctors.* Now the question becomes, what do you do with the information?

You make decisions. First, you get the proper tests. Then you choose one of three options: stimulate your own body's natural production, replace deficient hormones with bio-identical supplementation, or do both in combination. We'll first talk about boosting your own production. Then later we'll discuss replacement therapies.

Earlier we talked about using scientifically designed formulas or neutriceuticals for the purpose of stimulating, suppressing, or normalizing hormone function. In combination with improved diet and exercise, such products offer exceptional alternatives to the actual replacement of hormones. Depending on your age, health, and commitment level to following a structured regimen, this wellness alternative can work to improve FSH and LH production via the pituitary, stimulate estrogen and progesterone production, and improve both the balance and metabolism of female sex hormones.

Again, a proper evaluation of your endocrine system is necessary before making decisions about using any of these formulas. Tampering or attempting to alter your hormonal system without proper, objective lab results will most likely lead to further complications. Reviewing the earlier section, *Laboratory Methods and Testing,* should help.

Andropause—It's a "Guy" Thing

You didn't think I was going to leave you guys out, did you? I imagine a good number of you flipped directly to this section to get a quick glance at what help might be available to you. You can smile because science continues to look after our interests when it comes to maintaining our youthful bodies and drives. I'm not just implying an interest in sexual drive, but also confidence, ambition, and energy. Losing these often leads to the "girlie man" syndrome. Seriously, the decline of actively available androgens (testosterone) can be as devastating to a man as menopause is to a woman.

So, what exactly is *andropause?* It's the "professional" term for what people call "male menopause." Male menopause is a misnomer because men don't menstruate. Instead, they go through a gradual decline in their ability to produce sufficient levels of testosterone. At the same time, the estrogen-to-testosterone ratio also changes. Every man is affected differently by these changes and to different degrees. This is the reason that some men age with complete vitality, vigor, and virility, while others do not.

Up until recently, andropause was commonly overlooked because testosterone takes a slow and gradual dive compared to the sudden and abrupt changes that occur with menopause. Also, most men tend to avoid doctors or any tests that might reveal imperfections in their health. Many, I've noticed, simply dismiss the possibility that the loss of hormone balance could happen to them. It's almost as if this condition somehow means they might be lesser men. Whatever the reason, men have generally kept their problems to themselves and have somewhat fooled society into thinking there were no problems. I guess the astronomical success of the drugs Viagra® and Cialas® have let the cat out of the bag!

Andropause is usually seen in middle-to-older-aged men, but even men in their late 20's may have imbalances in their hormone physiology. In recent years, we have clinically seen an increase in the number of younger men with elevated estrogen levels. Author Dr. Malcolm Carruthers paints a good clinical picture:

> "The typical story is of a middle-aged man who loses his sex drive, strength, energy and enthusiasm for life and love. Action man has become inactive man. An all-enveloping mental and physical tiredness descends on him, often for no apparent reason. He changes from being a positive, bullish person who is good to be around, to a negative pessimistic, depressed bear with a sore head and is increasingly difficult to work with. At work, he is seen to have 'gone off the boil' and no amount of encouragement or urging improves his performance. At home, family relations tend to become increasingly strained, and social life and activities dwindle and wilt. His sexual life is usually a disaster area, with the loss of libido and intermittent failure to achieve an erection leading to performance anxiety and eventually complete impotence. This creates a downward spiral of failing function both in the bedroom and in the boardroom."[34]

Several underlying conditions result in andropause. These conditions affect primary andropause, secondary andropause, functional andropause, and genetic disorders. The most common type, functional andropause, takes place when the ratios between testosterone and other hormones shift out of balance. This typically occurs when the serum testosterone-to-estrogen level grows smaller. For example, a normal serum testosterone-to-estrogen ratio might be 50:1. Some men with andropause have ratios as low as 8:1. *In many cases, these men may show normal lab ranges of testosterone, but the relative estrogen dominance overwhelms the presence of normal testosterone levels.*

Attempting to correct this condition by increasing serum testosterone with the use of an exogenous form (intramuscular injection or cream) isn't a total solution. Estrogen levels will increase along with the higher levels of testosterone, resulting in the same low ratio. *Correcting functional andropause requires reducing or binding up excess estrogen.*

---

[34] *Maximizing Manhood,* Malcolm Carruthers, published by Harper Collins, 1997

It appears there's only a small decline in *total* blood testosterone throughout the lifespan. The problem is that total testosterone measures reflect both the protein-bound (inactive) form of testosterone *and* the free (active) form that's not bound to protein. In the past, little attention was given to isolated, <u>active</u>-testosterone patterns. Recent research has established, however, that as men age, their levels of free, active testosterone decrease significantly, while their levels of Sex Hormone Binding Globulin (SHBG) increase dramatically. In fact, the free fraction of testosterone contained in the total drops 1–2% per year while the SHBG fraction gains almost as much, leaving the total about the same.

But it's only the free fraction that keeps men "young"!

As free testosterone drops while bound testosterone increases, estrogen begins to dominate the free fraction. This causes most of the problems men experience as they age, *including prostate problems.*

A high estrogen condition highlights the importance of proper hormone testing as well as employing the knowledge to understand the findings. Too often I witness inadequate testing as I read the lab findings of male patients referred to me. In many cases they have been told that their testosterone levels are okay and there is nothing to worry about. So, they walk away with a sense of relief, thinking they are "still men." However, they also feel frustrated and confused as to why they don't feel the drive for living that they once did.

The average healthcare professional hasn't been well trained in identifying symptoms connected with andropause. Instead, the side effects of andropause such as high blood pressure, high cholesterol levels, and weight gain are treated as individual "diseases" without ever recognizing the single hormonal connection. Unfortunately, the managed-care health system doesn't look favorably upon the routine measurement of hormone levels for men who don't have serious hormonal dysfunction.

Andropause is becoming a serious health problem in industrialized countries. Many experts feel that this may be due to the increased levels of xenoestrogens and exotoxins in the environment,[35] the increased levels of stress placed on working individuals, the lack of essential fatty

---

[35] Vermeulen A., "Environmental, Human Reproduction, Menopause and Andropause." *Environmental Health Prospectives,* Supplement 1993;101:91-100

acids and nutrients in diets,[36] and the increased demands for hepatic (liver) detoxification placed upon us.

The Signs and Symptoms of Andropause

- Decrease in libido or desire for sex
- Decrease in spontaneous morning erections (most common early sign)
- Difficulty in maintaining or starting full erection
- Spells of mental fatigue and inability to concentrate
- A growing prostate and PSA level
- Depression
- Decreased initiative
- Muscle soreness
- Decrease in physical stamina
- Increase in total cholesterol or triglycerides
- Decrease in HDL cholesterol
- Elevation of fasting blood glucose
- Elevation in blood pressure
- Unexplained mid-section weight gain
- Increase in fat distribution in breast area or hips
- Development of varicose veins or hemorrhoids
- Changes in visual acuity

And, of course, the tendency toward prostate cancer is linked to the physiological changes of andropause.

Therefore, when testosterone levels are being measured, it's crucial to have the free fraction hormone levels measured as well as estrogen. Free-fraction testosterone can be measured in both saliva and serum.

---

[36] Linder MC, Nutrition and metabolism of fats. Nutritional Biochemistry and Metabolism. 2nd edition. Appleton and Lange, 1991:51-83

Types of Salivary Hormone Profiles Typically Used

I'm including some technical information here, but it gives you an idea of how we work to measure the effects of hormone changes in both men and women, and how replacement support is brought into play.

- ❑ **Adrenal Salivary Index (ASI):** This test measures the circadian rhythm of cortisol in a single day. The test requires the patient to collect a sample of saliva in the morning, at noon, in the afternoon, and at bedtime. Measurements of cortisol, DHEA, SigA, and SigA gliadin proteins are reported.

- ❑ **Short Post Menopausal Panel (PHP 1):** This panel measures baseline hormone levels of estradiol, estriol, estrone, DHEA, testosterone, and progesterone from one random saliva specimen. It does not measure pituitary hormones LH and FSH. This type of test is appropriate to determine pre- and post-hormone levels after some type of hormone augmentation program is initiated.

- ❑ **Long Post Menopausal Panel (PHP 2):** This panel employs two saliva specimens in the following order: the first sample is random and used as a baseline for estradiol, estriol, estrone, progesterone, DHEA, and testosterone. For 5-7 days, a hormone challenge is given, i.e. a therapeutic trial of one or more hormones is instituted. The hormone challenge should reflect the estimated peak maintenance dosage to be used in a proposed treatment plan. The second sample is collected on day 6 or 7. All six hormones are measured again to assess the effect of the challenge.

- ❑ **Expanded Post Menopausal Hormone Panel (ePHP 1):** This test measures estradiol, estrone, estriol, progesterone, DHEA, testosterone, LH, and FSH. It's identical to the Short Post Menopausal panel, except it measures pituitary hormones. This profile allows the interpretation of the pituitary-ovarian axis. It's the most common and appropriate test when evaluating a patient who isn't taking hormone replacement therapy.

- ❑ **Pre Menopausal Female Hormone Profile (FHP):** This panel uses eleven saliva samples that are collected during specified time slots throughout the menstrual cycle. The profile maps the levels of progesterone and estradiol during the menstrual cycle. Testosterone and DHEA levels are also measured and calculated to reflect the average follicular, ovulatory, and luteal phases of the cycle. This is the most advanced and well-reported test available in the healthcare system today. This test is appropriate for women who are not menopausal and are having menstrual irregularities.

- ❑ **Male Hormone Profile (MHP):** This panel provides the measurements of testosterone, dihydrotestosterone, DHEA, progesterone, and estrone. It requires that the patient collect one saliva sample. This test is appropriate for males who are taking some type of exogenous hormone such as testosterone.

- ❑ **Expanded Male Hormone Profile (eMHP):** This test provides the same measurements of the MHP but also includes LH and FSH. This test provides a means to evaluate the pituitary-gonadal axis and should be used as a standard baseline in male patients.

Some wellness doctors are certified to help you with hormone rebalancing assessments along with well-tested therapies. Some therapies use natural supplementation (nutriceuticals) or *biologically identical hormones* (hormones identical to those already found in your body) to help bring about effective hormonal balance reminiscent of youth. For example, my rebalancing therapies are formulated to "mimic" the effects of natural body chemistry without causing the awful side effects often experienced with the use of pharmaceutical synthetic hormones.

The Role of Vitamin D in Health

I can't leave this chapter without telling you that one of the most powerful "neutriceuticals" that you can use for disease prevention is the pro-hormone, vitamin D, from sunlight. That's right, sunlight! For decades, the dominant myth has been to stay out of the sun to avoid skin cancer and early skin aging, and to slather ourselves with toxic sunscreens if we *must* be in the sun. But that advice has created an epidemic in vitamin D deficiencies across North America, an epidemic implicating common pathologies such as at least 17 varieties of cancer as well as diabetes, heart disease, stroke, hypertension, autoimmune diseases, depression, chronic pain, osteoarthritis, osteoporosis, muscle weakness, muscle wasting, birth defects, periodontal disease, and more. You need to do your own research on Vitamin D and *pay attention to the latest findings.* I recommend that you visit www.vitamindcouncil.org and www.mercola.com to find up-to-date articles covering the subject, including how to test if you need to. For the time being, I will quickly summarize what you need to know so you understand the opportunity missed by so many. You will need to do your research to get the details.

- An *Optimal* level of sunlight exposure (with suitable UV eye protection) is the *best* way to get your vitamin D levels into the healthful range. "Optimal" means that your skin never turns more than a *light* shade of pink from exposure. However, you must avoid burning at all costs. For sunlight, more is not better.

- If you live above 30 degrees north latitude, you probably *can't* get adequate sunlight exposure for about six months of each year. Other factors are also involved: clouds, pollution, altitude, skin pigmentation, and a person's age.

- Risk for the most serious form of skin cancer, melanoma, appears to actually *decrease* with optimal sunlight exposure.

- A high ratio of omega-6 to omega-3 oils in the diet seems to increase the risk of skin cancer from sunlight exposure.

- If you think you might need to supplement with Vitamin D3, work with a wellness doctor to start. Vitamin D is fat-soluble and can be toxic when dosed at high levels. However, overdosing from *sunlight exposure* is highly unlikely because of the body's self-regulating mechanisms.

- For those who decide to supplement with D3 (but not if you're predisposed to high blood calcium levels), the blood test to use is **25-hydroxyvitamin D. An optimal range appears to be 50–65 ng/ml (*much* higher than what is considered "normal.") This is the range found in *healthy* people in tropical and subtropical parts of the world receiving healthy levels of sun exposure. Make sure your testing lab uses the correct assay, DiaSorin.**

Okay, we're finished with the "hormone education" chapter. It should serve you well as you embark on new experiences in wellness practice and self-care. Now it's time to take a leap into the passion of wellness. You can think of the next two chapters as being the capstone on understanding the *Reclaim 24* lifestyle. These chapters may challenge your beliefs and habits. So get ready!

PART III:
ADOPTING A PASSION FOR WELLNESS

You need to know that *most* of the fault for any failures you might be having comes at the hands of the **BIG FIVE STRESS AGENTS:**

1. <u>**Big Myth**</u> **– Poor information** that continues to fool the public year after year, leading the unaware to poor choices about health, dieting, and fitness.

2. <u>**Big Medicine**</u> **– A "sickness care" system** that bills itself as "health care." Because it is so misused, traditional medicine has become the leading cause of death and injury in the U.S. (not cancer, not heart disease, not car accidents, and certainly not the bird flu or swine flu).

3. <u>**Big Pharma**</u> **– Huge pharmaceutical companies** interested in huge profits and <u>lifelong</u> <u>customers</u> who will deliver those profits day in and day out. Goal: Get people onto drugs as early as possible and keep them on those drugs as long as possible without intentionally killing them (lost profits).

4. <u>**Big FakeFoods**</u> **– The gigantic processed food industry** interested in—you guessed it—profit, profit, profit from selling its cheap, denatured, calorie-loaded, fat-dripping, trans-fat-impregnated, chemical-laden, and chemically addictive **counterfeit food products**. Your health and wellness are of little concern to Big FakeFoods despite its self-serving, deceptive claims to the contrary. Their products are slowly killing you … legally!

5. <u>**Big Chemistry**</u> **– The chemical industry** that poisons our environment, bloodstreams, and organs while supposedly making life more convenient for us. How well is it working?

15: The Leap from Disease Care to Wellness Care

Translation: "If you want wellness, you simply *must* change the beliefs and habits that keep you from being well."

Not too long ago, the Discovery Health Channel aired an episode of a woman who had been physically fit in the past, but through some life circumstances had allowed her health to slip. She gained over 100 pounds. One morning she woke up and realized she was a young woman living in an old woman's body.

She started to diet, exercise, and lift weights, and the pounds starting falling off. She was such an inspiration to her family that her husband and her parents decided to join her, and now they are all losing weight as well as gaining lean muscle and confidence. And there's another uplifting element, too; as you witness the positive changes in others whom you've helped, your self-image further strengthens and the cycle renews. This makes life very, very rich!

If you give the 12-week action plan an honest chance to alter some of the undesirable aspects of your life, you'll find your time and effort to be well spent. This program induces changes—both visible and not so visible. These changes result in greater joy and quality of life not only for you but for your family as well. The joy comes from making good choices both outwardly and within your imagination. The joy also comes from wonderful wellness benefits, including an enhanced self-image. But just as important if not more so, it's about being able to *be there,* with all you possess, for those who you love and who depend on you!

So far so good. And congratulations for being willing to read this far. You've taken the first step in learning more about this thing called "wellness." But I've got to tell you, there's yet a whole other dimension to wellness awaiting your exploration. The 12-week *Reclaim 24* Action Plan that I've laid out for you only begins to address it. It gives you a taste. The next dimension involves the giant leap from disease care to wellness care. It involves shattering the fiction that prevents maximum wellness—and there's plenty of fiction to be shattered! So please read on. I'll try to make the wellness topic more tangible, more accessible for

187

you so you can also understand the implications of *not* having maximum wellness in your corner. To put it most simply, I'm inviting you to adopt the same passion for wellness that has been my gift in this life. Perhaps you'll even adopt a passion for telling others about it, including who may spontaneously ask you about your secrets if you've been following the *Reclaim 24* Action Plan. And in the best of all worlds, you'll become a highly qualified wellness mentor!

* * *

Everyone needs to know the differences between a health-care system and a disease-care system. Also, why the two are so often confused in this country. Are you ready to look at those differences and how they can and do affect you? If you are able to keep an open mind, you'll be able to make much better choices about how to stay optimally healthy for life. You'll get much closer to that ideal. of having a body, mind, and emotions that brim with vitality.

NOTICE: If you're convinced a that a doctor's only purpose is to fix you up or make you feel better when something seems to be wrong, read no further. You are wasting your time.

In Chapter 1, I pointed out that the practice of maximum wellness can grow to about 95% self-care. That still holds. It means wellness is 95% about YOU and your willingness to do for yourself what doctors can't. Yet, fear of change often keeps people from pursuing a wellness lifestyle. Most will go to their grave without ever taking personal responsibility for their health. They would much rather have their "doctor authorities" take care of them and make all their key health—or sickness—decisions. There's not much one can say about that. It's a choice. It's certainly not for me. And it's not for those whom I coach and mentor in my practice. Where do you stand?

I'm now going to explain how your body works, how chiropractic works, and how drugs work. You'll learn that you don't have to depend on taking unnecessary, risky, and often terribly expensive medications every time you feel sick or feel a pain. And you'll learn that having parts of your body cut out of you because they've been diagnosed as being "diseased" is a rather strange way to build health! This knowledge is a paradigm shift for people who have cut their teeth on the principles of conventional medicine—and paradigm shifts shake people's worlds!

I'll explain why medical practice, with its drug foundation, isn't set up to help you in your quest for a life of *optimized wellness—*if wellness is what you want. So hang on to your hat. You could be in for an interesting ride! And if you're a baby-boomer, here's a chance to get more of that BOOM back into your life!

Symptoms: Your Body's Often-Delayed Wake-Up Calls

Let's start with a quick look at distress symptoms—the main barometer that the medical community and drug industry use to determine if you are sick, how sick you are, and how they will "treat" you! If you've adopted the mindset of traditional medicine, you think in terms of symptoms, too. That thinking permeates the entire subject of "medicine." Moreover, to be "treated" in the medical community seldom means being placed on the path to healing or wellness. Most often it means reducing or masking symptoms—often for life—and hoping you'll feel better in the interim. But the practice of wellness is something altogether different. It's not just about having less distress than you did at the outset, or about having blood test numbers look better.

Now don't get me wrong: *all* health restoration systems in the world rely on *some* types of signs or symptoms of abnormality or distress to identify what "corrections" must be applied to get us back into better balance. Many of these signs or symptoms in fact may not be associated with distress at all. What all the world's health restoration systems *don't* have in common is the medical penchant to mask or cover up symptoms rather than go deeper into the heart of what is creating the imbalance that brought on the symptoms in the first place. Repeating what I said in the last paragraph, sometimes these symptom cover-ups go on for life.

As an example of what it means to go deeper, if you're getting cavities in your teeth, it makes great sense to have them drilled and filled, especially if you're repairing them long before the cavities penetrate too deeply. That is common-sense pain and damage prevention, yes? But why in the world are you getting cavities in the first place? Why don't we answer *that* question?

See?

Filling cavities is covering up symptoms (holes in teeth) and won't prevent new ones from forming. That is disease care. In contrast, wellness care or practice is answering the question about why some people get cavities and others don't, and learning how to earn lifetime membership in the *second* club.

As you know, we experience different types of physical, emotional, and mental symptoms of distress when things are not right with our bodies. Stub a toe or cut your finger and your symptoms instantly tell you something is wrong. Further, you pretty much know what to do about it: let out a screech or fetch a Band-Aid. More serious problems often require the emergency care that modern medical practitioners are so skilled at providing. After all, we do need great surgeons to save the lives of those suffering from trauma or physical birth defects. Some people genuinely benefit from cosmetic surgery, for example, and I'm not just talking about silicone implants. Some dental patients really do benefit from oral surgery when things have deteriorated too far. There are many other examples where surgery plays a legitimate and helpful role. No one can dispute that.

But did you know that ...

- ❑ **A cavity usually develops for two years before it begins to hurt?**

- ❑ **Cancer usually doesn't hurt at all until the end stages?**

- ❑ **Nearly half of the people who have heart attacks in America get no prior warning symptoms? That the first indication something is wrong is their funeral bill?**

So, why in the world do so many people who *do not* need critical care put themselves into the hands of "healthcare" systems that rely so much on reacting to and "treating" symptoms of distress? Doesn't it make more sense to look deeper to eliminate the conditions—*the causes*—that lead to the symptoms of disease, illness, or infirmity, long before those symptoms arise (if they arise at all)? Of course it does. But the public has been duped about the meaning of healthcare for many years. Thankfully, times are changing.

Most people have come to equate health with not being sick, and not being sick with the absence of distress symptoms. The reason for this thinking is the mindset of those who practice medicine—the currently predominant system of "healthcare" in this country. This system is commonly called the allopathic model of treatment. It's the "conventional medicine" with which we are all so familiar.

190

The Allopathic Model: Brilliant for Crisis or Emergencies

The allopathic model (allopathy) is the "healing" method practiced by physicians who graduate from medical school and who write *M.D.* after their names. Whenever you see the adjective "medical," it's the allopathic model that is being referred to, e.g., "American *Medical* Association." By definition, the allopathic model fosters the early detection and correction of symptoms, disease, and infirmity. The best you can usually hope for is early detection through screening and such. Typically you have to wait until you get sick or diseased before conventional medicine can "kick in" to help you.

But if you have to wait for something negative to happen, doesn't it make more sense to call this "sick care" rather than "health care?" If you're not sure, keep reading. All will become clear.

Q: What Stands between Sick Care and Health Care?
A: Drugs, Surgery, and Their Checkered Reputations.

Here are three, life-altering things you need to know about the allopathic model:

1. Respected scientific studies[37] show clearly that <u>THE AMERI-CAN MEDICAL SYSTEM IS THE LEADING CAUSE OF DEATH AND INJURY IN THE UNITED STATES</u>. Not cancer, not heart disease, not car accidents, and certainly not the bird flu or swine flu.

2. An increase in the supply of medical doctors in a geographic region is linked to an increase in population mortality (people die earlier).

3. When hospitals go on strike, the morbidity and mortality rates go down (fewer people get sick or die during strike periods).

Those, my friends, are the seldom talked about "side effects" of our allopathic "healthcare" model. Do you see something strange in that picture?

---

[37] Nutrition Institute of America article, "Death by Medicine," authored by Gary Null, Ph.D., Carolyn Dean, M.D., N.D., Martin Feldman, M.D., Debora Rasio, M.D., and Dorothy Smith, Ph.D.

Well, just about everybody knows the allopathic model is brilliant when emergency or disease care is needed, but it has much less to offer those who seek true health care, disease prevention, or wellness. On the contrary, folder upon folder of reliable statistics show that...

> ## "When you apply sick care to people who need health care, you get more sick and dead people."

Here are three jaw-dropping facts:

1. At least three jumbo jets worth of people are dying every day in America because of medical errors and adverse drug reactions. *That's three jumbo jets full of people just falling out of the sky (some think the real numbers may be twice that).*

2. The chance of dying in an aviation accident is one in two million. The chance of dying of a medical accident is one in 200.

3. Each year 16,000 people die from using NSAIDS (non-steroidal inflammatory drugs) such as Advil™. In contrast, 10,000 people a year die from using illicit drugs such as crack, cocaine, and so on. But we don't hear about the 16,000 people dying from NSAIDS. Or the two million people addicted to prescription drugs. Why do you suppose that is?

Once again, the public is being duped. The allopathic model isn't working as a *healthcare* system. Drugs and surgery are being radically overused because an emergency or trauma-treatment system is trying to serve as a healthcare system. **But when the #1 killer in a society is the healthcare system itself, that system is failing to protect you.**

The Wellness Model: An Oasis for Self-Responsible People

Wellness practice goes far beyond pursuing the absence of symptoms, disease, and infirmity. It's an on-going day-to-day and moment-to-moment stress-reduction lifestyle. It's a lifestyle that requires taking personal responsibility and making smart, healthy choices with each chance you get (or at least with the vast majority of chances that you get since perfection isn't simple). The wellness model promotes individual well-being through balancing the following personal areas: physical, emotional, intellectual, and spiritual. I covered this in Chapter 2.

192

Okay, back to the wellness model of healthcare. It's based on the principle of maintaining optimum health by preventing or reducing opportunities for disease and infirmity to take hold. It also allows the body's innate healing intelligence to contribute to that prevention in the best ways possible. This model wants to *remove the causes* that lead to unnecessary[38] symptoms of distress and not just cover them up.

In the disease care or allopathic model, you are *moving away* from something you do not want: disease, symptoms of distress, infirmity, death. In the wellness model, you're *moving toward* something you want: greater ability to heal yourself, greater well-being, better digestion, better function, better quality of life. The joy of living!

The allopathic model, based on fear, endeavors to move patients away from pain. Disease is considered to be the presence of something evil. The wellness model, on the other hand, isn't based on fear. It's based on empowerment. In this model, disease is considered to be the absence of something good, something essential. What can we do to remedy that absence?

A Questionable Reward for Serving English Royalty!

When British seamen used to come home from war with their skin falling off and their teeth falling out (scurvy), the "authorities" got rid of the "evil spirits" that had overtaken the seamen by burning the men at the stake. That approach obviously worked to destroy those nasty spirits because once the men were toasted, spreading of the affliction was stopped in its tracks! What more proof could you ask for? Very smart, those royal consultants!

But James Lind finally discovered that it wasn't the presence of evil spirits at all that caused those seamen to come home with their skin falling off and their teeth falling out, but the absence of something good, something essential: Vitamin C. The disease disappeared once seamen ate limes while at sea (and so they became known as "limeys"). Or maybe we're all wrong about that. Maybe someday we'll discover that Vitamin C scares away evil spirits, just as garlic wards off vampires.

Today, body parts considered cancerous are also burned with drugs and radiation, or excised with surgery. If a patient dies from a caustic

---

[38] Some symptoms of distress, such as nausea, are desirable because they may be telling you something important!

cancer treatment as so many do, well, that's the way things go. At least that infernal evil has been destroyed! Some things never change.

And one more thing. Drugs place tremendous stress upon the body, even when they are acting the way they are intended to act with few if any notable side effects. In this respect, drugs and *wellness* practice are incompatible. Yet, sometimes drugs are necessary. So you do, indeed, want to keep yourself in the greatest state of wellness that you can in order to handle the stress of drugs if they should become necessary.

> *All medicines, in a way, are poisons—you try to poison the disease before you poison the patient. That goes for aspirin or anything else we take.*
>
> –David Spodic, M.D.,
> Professor of Medicine
> University of Massachusetts

Look. This purpose of this book isn't to bash the many wonderful medical doctors who are no less dedicated to helping interested people than I am. Some of my best friends are M.D.s. Rather, **I'm challenging the fact that our country's disease care model is called healthcare—and people actually believe it!** With this *disease care model* in place, M.D.s have an almost impossible job. They don't have the right tools or the right premise to deliver *healthcare*. Moreover, they have the AMA and Big Pharma breathing down their necks to "toe the line." So, they are equipped to "treat" disease and its symptoms, but seldom the deeper causes. And woe unto him or her who gets too creative or who questions the soundness of current medical practice as dictated by medical and pharmaceutical "authorities."

* * *

Although allopathy is still referred to as "conventional" medicine, alternatives for *true* healthcare stand right before our eyes. Notable among these is wellness-oriented chiropractic. That's my specialty for supporting nervous-system health. Let's take a look at it.

194

Innate Intelligence: Where Healing Really Comes from

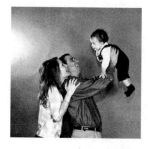

Have you ever seen a bored newborn? Of course not. Babies radiate awe, joy, wonder, vitality, energy, life, and rejuvenation. It's their natural state. But it's your natural state, too! You are always in touch with the magic of life. Even the most ill person retains a healing ability: cut their skin, and they'll bleed and begin healing. If there's life, there's still a spark of healing, of hope.

Chiropractors have neither the interest nor lawful authority to put "invasion chemicals" into your body that we call drugs. Nor do we slice anything out of you with surgery. Instead, we release an often-serious form of stress that locks itself in your spine between various vertebra. It's a stress that prevents you from functioning at your best.

Vertebral stress points in your spine can choke off the nerves that regulate your immune system, digestive system, and elimination system. In fact, all your body systems. These nerves enable communication among all organs, tissues, and cells of your body. If you have stress points in your spine that are choking off nerves, you simply cannot function at your physical, emotional, and mental best.

Chiropractors correct or release vertebral stress using professional techniques called spinal adjustments. For over a century, people who have suffered from all kinds of

> "Inside your body is a wonderful pharmacy. You name it, the human body can make it—tranquilizers, sleeping pills, anti-cancer drugs; the right dose at the right time for the right organ with no side effects. All the instructions you need come with the packaging which is your Innate Intelligence."
>
> – Deepack Chopra, M.D., world-renowned and best-selling author and Harvard-trained Endocrinologist

conditions and who were told to "learn to live with it" have found a return to health under chiropractic care. And yet, chiropractors don't "treat" disease; *they remove barriers to health.* They help release blockages between you and the miraculous life force always striving to flow through and heal you. They empower you to be healthy!

Now for a little deeper look into chiropractic principles, processes, and practices. I'll start by answering the question, *What Is Innate Intelligence?*

Dr. Lewis Thomas, M.D., said, "...a kind of super intelligence exists in each of us, infinitely smarter and possessed of technical know-how far beyond our present understanding." This is your *innate intelligence,* the inborn wisdom of your body. It's the intelligence that allows your body to constantly adapt to its ever-changing environments. For example, this intelligence keeps your heart beating. It knows how to digest your food after you've eaten, without your having to think about it. It heals a cut on your finger (no, your Band-Aid doesn't do the healing). And it kicks your immune system into high-gear when your body is being invaded by bacteria.

Innate intelligence resides everywhere in your body. It is mediated by your brain, which communicates with every muscle, gland, organ, and cell in your body via your nervous system. Chiropractors are the only doctors, as a profession, who *formally* recognize the body's inborn wisdom or intelligence. They work on and with the body so that our innate intelligence can express itself as near to 100% as possible. And that's where the practical foundations of chiropractic come in.

Why Chiropractic Works to Keep Your Nervous System Healthy

Chiropractic is based upon four crucial principles. Here they are:

1. **Your Body is a Self-Healing and Self-Regulating Organism.**

2. **Your Nervous System is Under "Computer" Control.**

3. **Interferences in the Nervous System Create Health Problems.**

4. **Your Spine is the Most Likely Place for Nervous System Interference to Occur.**

Here's what each of these four principles means to you.

    1. **Your Body is a Self-Healing, Self-Regulating Organism.**
This means your body was designed to heal itself. Did you know that approximately every 30 days you get a brand new liver? Over the period of a month, your liver cells die off and are replaced by new ones. Every four months all of your blood cells are replaced. And before the end of the year, about 90% of you

is new—at least physically! This process continues year after year for your entire life. Awesome! The point is that your body is in a constant mode of change and repair. However, to do this it must follow an exact program that was set in motion almost from the time you were conceived. So, if you're not well, it stands to reason that your body is unable to follow the program for some reason.

2. **Your Nervous System is Under "Computer" Control.** In order for your body to follow its self-healing program, there needs to be communication from point to point. Your nervous system, the master control network of your body, orchestrates this communication at the physical level.[39] Your nervous system is made up of your brain, spinal cord, and spinal or peripheral nerves—the nerves that extend from your spine to every area of your body. Your brain is the control center—or at least mediator—of literally every function in your body. If your brain dies, you die. As long as your brain can effectively communicate with every organ, tissue, cell, nook, and cranny, your body has the opportunity to be at its very best health. This condition of unfettered communication is what we should think of as "being normal."

3. **Interferences in the Nervous System Create Health Problems.** Your brain sends 100% of your body's information and energy down your spinal cord. Your spinal cord is protected by 24 movable vertebrae. Spinal nerves exit between these vertebrae and go out to deliver the messages sent from your brain, through your spine, to each muscle, gland, and organ— and ultimately to every cell of your body. And through the same system, messages are returned. As long as there is no functional interference in your spinal cord and spinal nerves, your body has the ability to receive messages from and return messages to the brain so that you can function at your best. In other words, as close to 100% as possible when all things are taken into consideration.

---

[39] There appear to be other, higher-order communication functions going on among body, mind, and emotions that may extend beyond the physical nervous system, but that's a subject I can't cover in this book.

But if nerve restrictions suppress or garble these messages, your body is not able to do what it was programmed to do—heal itself. It is not *able* to follow or execute its built-in, self-healing program. But there's even more to know that so few people do. In a new book, Dr. James Chestnut discusses how the most recent, unquestionable research shows that *changing the way the spine moves actually alters the form, function, and structure of the brain!* Further, spinal movement literally charges the brain's "batteries" and allows it to fully function. In fact, movement of the spine generates 90% percent of the stimulation and nutrition to the brain.[40] *Reduce spinal movement through restrictions or inactivity and the brain can no longer receive full power and can no longer function correctly.*

4. **Your Spine is the Most Likely Place for Nervous System Interference to Occur.** If your spinal vertebrae are compressed or get out of alignment, even slightly (which injuries, poor posture, and many other life stressors can do to you), the resulting stress points can <u>act as resistors</u> to the distribution of your nervous system energy and impulses and diminish your body's ability to stay healthy. When a vertebral stress point chokes a spinal nerve, it only takes a pressure <u>as light as the weight of a quarter</u> for three minutes to reduce the function of that nerve by 60%. Moreover, degenerative changes in the nerve, itself, begin to take place within three hours[41].

My responsibility as a Doctor of Chiropractic (D.C.) is to locate stress-creating misalignments or compressions in your spine. Then I gradually coax the vertebrae back into place so that normal nerve and structural function is restored and other damaged, inflamed tissues in the region can begin to heal (also a necessity). This allows the nervous system to once again effectively communicate and control bodily functions. Greater health is the result.

Why Treating Symptoms Can't Help Us Restore Health

Because the medical and pharmaceutical cultures have influenced this country for so long, most people judge their health based on the presence or absence of symptoms—usually distress symptoms. This is how the

---

[40] Dr. Roger Sperry, Nobel Prize Winner for Brain Research
[41] Dr. Suh, University of Colorado neurophysiologist

medical and drug industries think. It's how they expect *you* to think. However, as you read earlier, symptoms are often the *last* sign your body gives you to tell you something is wrong. It's like having termites. They silently work behind the scenes to destroy your home's infrastructure. You're oblivious to the hidden damage until something starts to crumble (a symptom). Only then do you begin to understand the full extent of the damage that's taken place in the dark.

That's why waiting for symptoms to appear is just about the worst way to fend for your health and your family's health. Symptoms are just the tip of the iceberg—signs that *something* has already gone wrong. And the most disappointing thing about symptoms is you often don't know what the *real* problem is or how long it's been incubating (most cancers incubate 10 years before they are detectable).

Take headaches for instance. Headaches can have an incredible number of underlying causes. Taking aspirin for headaches might relieve the distress symptoms, but the headaches will just come back if you don't remove their causes (and if you don't also make sure your body is in the best condition to heal itself of any damage that's been done in the meantime). If you fail to act, whatever is causing headaches may continue to do more damage. Before long, just having headaches might seem like a walk in the park! That's why wellness-chiropractic care—*the type that gets to deeper causes*—makes so much sense.

> *Research is revealing what many chiropractic patients have known for decades: they are healthier. 2,818 chiropractic patients filled out extensive surveys before, at the beginning of, and during chiropractic care. Significant improvements in quality of life, physical health, and mental/emotional health were revealed. They also reported decreased stress and increased life enjoyment. The benefits became evident as early as 1–3 months under care and showed continuing improvement as long as patients stayed under care. There was no apparent plateau, meaning the more chiropractic, the more the benefit.*
>
> –Blanks RHI, Schuster TL. A retrospective assessment of network care using a survey of self-rated health, wellness and quality of life. JVSR. 1997;1(4).

Heartburn is another common example. Recent TV drug commercials have told us that we can get 24-hour relief from heartburn just by taking one Nexium Purple Pill™ a day (a $6 billion/year business for the AstraZeneca drug company). Imagine that! But that's not part of any program for wellness, is it? Drugs just create more stress that your body has to deal with!

So, why are you getting heartburn in the first place? What's the cure? The cause is still there—possibly getting worse—and the side effects of the drug might even add to your misery. Just listen to what the commercials have to tell you about the drug's side effects! In fact, a recent study by the American Gastroenterological Association states that when healthy people discontinue proton pump inhibitors such as Nexium after eight weeks of use, users tend to get a rebound effect that makes acid secretion even worse. So back to the Purple Pill again? Or a substitute? Big Pharma would love that.

The Benefits of Regular, Preventative Chiropractic Care

Surely, vertebral stress points aren't the only causes of disease. Yet, if you have other things going on with you that are promoting disease or stress, you want the most benefit that your nervous system can deliver to deal with those things. Removing vertebral stress through regular chiropractic care allows your nervous system to keep functioning at its highest, self-healing level. That's a big part of wellness practice!

Indeed, regular care helps to prevent problems from developing in the first place—like headaches, acid stomachs, and dozens of other illnesses or chronic conditions. Just as brushing and flossing your teeth helps prevent tooth decay and gum disease, maintaining a healthy, strong spine prevents all the physical problems in your body that result from a spine that is losing integrity and movement; and with those losses, the ability to transmit nerve messages and power your brain. **Regular care is a smart, proactive way to keep your precious body working as designed.** It's not the only factor for staying well for sure, but it sets a stable foundation for you. It "raises the bar" for wellness.

The "Side Effects" of Chiropractic Care

One who indulges in preventative chiropractic care needs to be prepared to handle its side effects. These may include increased energy, improved digestion and elimination, disappearance of gastric reflux, blood sugar stabilization, easier weight control, better appearance, diminished allergies, improved immunity, and an uplifted mood. These are typical offshoots from using chiropractic to address your initial complaints of headaches, neck and back pain, numbness, or extremity pain. Are you ready to handle such side effects?

200

When Regular Chiropractic Care Might Not Help

Regular chiropractic visits might not benefit you all that much if you have no emotional stress in your life; if you stand, sit, and sleep with perfect posture; if you are not subject to harmful chemicals in the food you eat, the air you breathe, or the water you drink; if your diet and exercise programs are world class (which they will be if you follow my program); and if injuries are behind you. Do you know anybody like that? I didn't think so.

Your body goes into a defensive posture when you are injured or when life's many forms of stress reach a higher level than your energy and healing reserves can handle. Vertebral stress points occur as a result. Most often you are not able to feel them when they first arise (just like the beginnings of diseases). But as you've already learned, vertebral stress points choke off the life energy that must flow through your nervous system to keep you healthy. This, in turn, makes your body less able to handle stress, which creates even further stress in your spine. It's a no-win, cyclic affair that leads to a downward spiral in your health.

> *Did you know that only 10% of your nervous system is sensory? This means you can be feeling "fine" in that 10% while things are going haywire in the other 90% where you can't feel it! In such cases, "stories" relayed by vertebral stress points can become your best friend.*

A vertebral stress point often tells a story to a chiropractor. Every now and then, one will recur despite continued efforts at spinal readjustment. This happens, for example, when a distressed organ sends messages to the brain that the organ is not functioning well. The spine picks up the distress signals as they pass through it, and innately reacts by setting up a stress point at the specific vertebra where the nerves direct themselves to the distressed organ. This stress "symptom" is a good thing because it delivers a message to your doctor that otherwise might be missed. After all, local pain is often not present when organs are distressed.

The "Path of Indifference" Has Costs

The most important thing to remember about a vertebral stress point is that, left unattended, it slowly but surely damages nerves—along with the associated vertebrae and surrounding tissues that provide spinal support and function. The longer left unattended (waiting for distress to arise), the greater the impact on your health and well-being. Travel too far down the "path of indifference" and just releasing a vertebral stress no longer solves a problem by itself. A longer term of healing becomes necessary to get the support structure and peripheral tissues back to health. <u>Sometimes a total return to bone and tissue health is no longer even possible. Then drugs and the surgeon's knife may be the only answer.</u> I see this all too often in my practice. It's sad. IT DOESN'T HAVE TO BE THIS WAY. Surgery and parts replacement are fine if you are over the hill, <u>but why go over the hill long before your time?</u> And why pay the huge costs in pain, suffering, and dollars that go with it? What kind of quality of life is that?

The Benefits of Acute Chiropractic Care

You need acute care when you have pain or other forms of symptomatic discomfort. As you've learned from what you've just read, you can often avoid the need for acute care with *regular* chiropractic care—which, unlike drug use, is <u>truly</u> preventative. Regular care allows your innate healing intelligence to operate at its best to help prevent you from ever getting to the point of discomfort or disease in the first place. It removes obstacles.

But life happens. Even under the best of circumstances, various stressors or injuries can leave you with pain or discomfort—in your neck, spine, or elsewhere. Such discomfort often benefits from support and care beyond what your innate healing intelligence can provide, especially if that innate intelligence has been hampered by vertebral stress points for some time. Spinal adjustments can, and usually do, relieve some or all of this discomfort. But if you still need pain relief, a chiropractor is usually able to recommend a non-invasive relief approach for you. Please remember this, however:

> ## A symptom of distress usually disappears *long* before the *cause* of that symptom is eliminated.

You typically need a series of adjustments to make sure your spinal corrections "take hold" and your brain and nervous system are retrained to fully support your body's innate healing functions. <u>Each adjustment serves as an incremental step toward achieving your optimum level of wellness.</u> This approach works much the same way that orthodontic braces work to correct crooked teeth: continuous nudging over time.

Certainly not overnight! So, just as braces slowly shift teeth to their desired positions over a period of time, coaxing the spine to its best configuration, step by step, is seldom an immediate process. You need to be patient because it takes time to shift your physical infrastructure to a more healthful configuration and also *retrain* the parts of your nervous system to accept that shift. Muscles, ligaments, tissues, spinal nerves, <u>and brain</u>, must slowly conform or adapt, just as misaligned teeth with their connecting gums, ligaments, and nerves conform to the persistent influence of dental braces.

* * *

Do try to find a wellness-oriented chiropractor (in contrast to a short-term-pain-relief practitioner) who can support you with your personal wellness efforts. Any chiropractor worth his or her salt will provide you with adequate, one-on-one "interview" time or at least printed materials that allow you to get answers to questions about what type of chiropractic the doctor practices. You want your doctors to be compatible with you and your self-care interests in wellness.

In the next chapter, I'll talk more about how to choose a wellness doctor, even if not a chiropractor. I'll also tell you how I practice to give you additional ideas about what to look for in a wellness practitioner. As you expand your wellness I.Q., choosing the right doctors or consultants becomes easier, especially if you "network" with others who practice wellness.

A Final Note about Chiropractic

Many people wonder about the level of education that chiropractors receive. Chiropractic college provides more hours of classroom education than medical college (4,800 hours vs. 4,667 hours). On average, chiropractic students receive 200 more hours in anatomy, and 60 more hours in physiology than medical students do. Further, training in diagnosis is 630 hours vs. 324 hours, neurology 320 hours vs.112 hours, and orthopedics 210 hours vs. 156 hours. I'll let the numbers speak for themselves.

Everyone needs "hands-on" professional support to maintain maximum wellness levels, even wellness professionals. Please don't forget that. Yet, I also teach you how to *practice* wellness as part of your lifestyle. And I teach you that this practice is up to **95% *self-care***.

Self-care is not drudgery or destructive discipline when it's handled in the right ways. It is pampering! I show you how to pamper yourself with esteem-building exercise, foods that nourish, heal, and taste good, and stress-fighting habits that promote "ageless" living. Indeed, *Reclaim 24* is a pampering lifestyle if there ever was one, not a deprivation lifestyle. What good is "ageless living" if you have to be miserable doing the living? Few people can tolerate such misery for long, and they don't.

16: Pulling It All Together

Do you remember the story from Chapter 15 that described how British seamen contracted scurvy because they were missing vitamin C in their diets? In truth, a deficit in wellness—often accompanied by a ride on the Conveyor Belt to a Living Hell—is the product of all kinds of things missing from our lives. It's also a product of things that we add to our lives that don't belong there.

To repeat what I've said before, the practice of maximum wellness requires about 95% self-care. But the remaining 5% exceeds most of our capacities. Few if any of us know enough about the healing arts to render 100% self-care, no matter how proactive we are. Life happens! Even doctors are silly to treat themselves. You've heard the old cliché: "A doctor who treats himself has a fool for a patient." So if we're smart, we will work with one or more licensed professionals to complement our self-care wellness efforts. And how might we go about doing that?

Embracing the "Five Pillars of Optimized Health"

At the end of Chapter 3, I introduced the *Five Pillars of Optimized Health* that I've identified from studying, practicing, and teaching wellness, and which have become the foundation for *Reclaim 24*. I've found that these five areas cover most of the *proactive, preventative, holistic measures* that wellness professionals use to support their patients. When a wellness seeker visits my center, I assess the level of wellness he or she has achieved with respect to these five pillars. I'll repeat them here:

> Nervous System (from a structural, stress-release perspective)
> Organs and Glands (from a hormonal, nutritional perspective)
> Detoxification
> Nutrition
> Fitness/Motion/Exercise

Novice wellness seekers probably can't or shouldn't assess all these areas alone—at least not at the outset. They really do require the services of wellness professionals. As time goes on, however, continually learning about and monitoring your progress in each of the five areas works wonders. It helps you mentally focus on the purpose of your 5% professional support so you can keep moving toward your personal wellness potential. In the beginning, you might need a great deal more professional support than "5%"—at least until the wellness bug bites you and you "catch the wave" for high-energy surfing!

In any case, let's now take stock of what we've covered up to this point so you can recognize the roles that the five pillars play in your wellness lifestyle. Likewise, so that you are able to intelligently assess how well your wellness doctor, or prospective wellness doctor, is truly engaging in comprehensive wellness practice and not some lesser or limited form of support.

To begin with, if you have been following the *Reclaim 24*, 12-Week Action Plan (Part II of this book), you will already be far along the path to achieving wellness in the nutritional and the fitness/motion/exercise areas (pillars 4 and 5). You may be able to get along with little mentoring or professional support unless you really want to apply the five pillars to your full potential. Many people do. But your *progress* in those two areas can easily be limited, halted, or even reversed if your nervous system, organs, and glands are not functioning at their best—or if toxins are building up in your system and creating stress overload. So where do we stand with respect to pillars 1, 2, and 3?

I already covered nervous system support from a structural perspective in the last chapter, "The Leap from Disease Care to Health Care." There I talked about the importance of spinal health and movement to enable innate healing and brain charging. Of course, I also talked about the difference between disease care and health care, and how the practice of wellness is compatible with the latter. Read and understand that chapter and you will know more about the foundations of health than 10,000 people around you, and probably many more. You will also have a blueprint to help you choose wellness professionals.

In Chapters 13 and 14, I talked at length about the role of organ and gland health from a hormonal perspective. Once again, if you take the time to understand what those chapters are trying to tell you, you will be miles ahead of what you previously understood about wellness. Strangely, you will also be miles ahead of what most doctors understand!

The only component for achieving optimized health that I have yet to talk about in detail is detoxification. I'll do so now so that you have at least an introductory, educational closure to all five of the *Reclaim 24* pillars of optimized health. And if you've been following the *Reclaim 24*

Action-Plan blueprint, you will have some solid wellness practice under your belt.

Detoxify to Reduce and Handle Stress More Effectively

As with the term "wellness," "detoxification" (or "detoxing") has also become somewhat of a buzzword. I'll try to clarify some of the ideas behind detoxification because you can't practice maximum wellness without knowing a lot about it. That's why it's one of my five pillars for optimized health.

Few people, it seems to me, have been inspired to think this idea through, but the word "detoxification" in common use tends to have five different shades of meaning. These shades are usually jumbled together until mental confusion arises and people begin to talk past each other (do I sound too cynical?) In practice, "detoxification" takes on one or more of the following meanings in most people's minds:

1. **A bodily process in which toxins (unhealthy substances or molecules), are converted into less harmful or harmless substances and excreted.** The liver is our body's main detoxification and filtering organ, while the colon, kidneys, gallbladder, lungs, skin, blood, and lymphatic system serve (in part) to escort waste products and unhealthy substances out of the body. The general principle is that the liver, among its hundreds of functions, tries to convert harmful substances in the blood to less harmful or innocuous substances before sending them on their way to be eliminated or even reused.

2. **A process in which the body attempts to achieve a new homeostasis[42] after some hopefully positive change is made in diet or other behavior.** For example, quitting coffee requires a chemical rebalance in the body after caffeine—which was playing an addictive molecular role with cell receptors—is withdrawn. There are no "toxins" released to speak of, but one can sure feel lousy while the body's chemistry readjusts itself to live in the absence of the chemical stimulant. Alcohol and drug withdrawals

---

[42] Homeostasis is the body's natural tendency to maintain—or attempt at maintaining—an internal stability or balance. The organ systems of the body coordinate biological responses that automatically compensate for environmental changes.

are other examples that can have more potent side effects— and even dangers—as a new homeostasis is set into motion.

3. **An approach that intends, at least in the short term, to relieve stress on the liver and excretory organs so that they can better function at their jobs.** This approach tends to remove barriers to the body's ability to heal itself. There are many theories—some good, many not so good—related to "cleansing diets" and "cleansing agents" that a wellness practitioner must sort through before finding his or her best approach (when needed). There's a lot of myth and bad information out there to sort through. But again, this category of "detoxification" has to do with relieving stress on organs so they can function better and not directly with removing toxins.

4. **The avoidance or reduction of environmental toxins that come from food, drink, and air.** Of course, you can also absorb toxins through forms of physical contact other than food, drink, and air. As well, certain types of radiation can have toxic effects on your body. Awareness, reduction, and avoidance play large roles in preventing toxins from entering your system in the first place.

5. **The reduction or avoidance of emotional or mental stress.** This is one of the sneakier ways to "detox," but we know that emotional and mental stress have negative physical effects on the body that can lead to real toxins developing; or to organs losing their ability to carry out their detoxification roles efficiently; or to our genes expressing themselves in harmful ways.

Where Do Toxins Come From?

Toxins typically come from the world outside of us. They create physiological stress. However, mental and emotional stress can also lead to toxic body conditions, as I just mentioned. As well, normal metabolic processes can leave toxic residues behind if the liver and other excretory organs are not working up to speed. Simply put, our external and internal world has become a hazardous wasteland in which we must breathe polluted air, drink chemically polluted and "treated" water, eat processed and altered foods devoid of all nutrition (or worse), take daily medications and synthetic hormones, and react to daily stress that is part of our culture or personal beliefs. Although technology and industrial advancement have led to wonderful improvements in our lives, they have also dramatically increased the presence of toxins. Now, our country is experiencing growing incidences of cancer, diabetes, high blood pressure, viruses, Alzheimer's, and virtually all other chronic and degenerative diseases.

What Have I Been Doing Wrong?

Most people experience significant toxin accumulation, detoxification insufficiencies, and suboptimal homeostasis conditions due to the content of their diets. The average American diet can render the liver sluggish so that it can no longer do its detoxification job well at all. The gallbladder can also become sluggish, if not clogged. This prevents certain wastes from being eliminated through the biliary system.

The stomach can no longer digest food as it should because enzyme and acid levels degrade. The small intestine loses some ability to absorb the proper nutrients. Sometimes it even allows substances to reenter the bloodstream that shouldn't. And the large intestine (colon) slows down, leading to constipation, irritable bowel syndrome, and other diseases. Add in large quantities of sugar-laden foods and drinks, artificial sweeteners, heavy metals in our air, food, and water supply, prescription and over-the-counter medications, and the average American body becomes a wonderful harbor for toxin build-up!

And here's the clinker: Genetically, the liver cannot recognize many offending, environmental substances to be the poisons that they are. Therefore, they don't get converted to less noxious substances or removed from the blood except by chance (over many years). They simply sneak through the liver's natural screening process and accumulate in the bones, fat, and other tissues, unrecognized for what they are. Then they slowly kill us, or poison our systems so that they cannot work properly. This generally means a lower quality of life.

In the meantime, the chemical industry and its regulatory minions say it's okay to have these thousands of chemical substances swimming in our bloodstreams and lodged in our tissues! Fluoride in drinking water is one example. Its molecules displace iodine, leading to a weakened thyroid function and more than a hundred other, well-documented health issues. It gets ugly. There are some very revealing books out there discussing the fluoride topic.

Another example is mercury. It can mimic or cause just about any illness currently known, or at least contribute to it.

Along these lines, it's important to understand that if you're deficient in essential metals or minerals, your body employs toxic, heavy metals to serve as "stand-ins." For example:

- Lead will replace calcium and deposit itself primarily in bone, disrupting the formation of red blood cells. Lead also contributes to poor bone health such as osteopenia and osteoporosis.

- Cadmium will replace zinc and tend to accumulate heavily in your kidneys. Cadmium overload is associated with peripheral neuropathy.

- Aluminum will replace magnesium and will, among other things, induce neurochemical changes. Aluminum has also been identified as a contributing factor to developing Alzheimer's.

- Nickel, which is carcinogenic, will replace manganese.

So, you do need to make sure you're getting vital nutrients in your diet in order to avoid toxic metals slipping in and taking over.

A third example is the grease-resistant coatings of perfluorinated chemicals on paper products such as french fry boxes, popcorn boxes, candy bar wrappers, hamburger wrappers, carryout bags, pizza boxes, and hundreds of other food items. Yes, these Dupont-developed coatings keep grease stains from developing (wow, what an advance), but the coatings also leach into food and are now found in the bloodstreams of 96% of all Americans as well as wildlife in the most unexpected parts of the world. The chemicals even penetrate placentas to contaminate a fetus before birth. What's worse, when in the blood, the chemicals convert to likely human carcinogens C8 and PFOA—compounds that Dupont uses to make Teflon.

As wellness practitioners, we need to think about how to avoid or reduce our exposure to such chemicals—that is when we are even allowed to know about their presence or toxicity without whistle-blowers first speaking up and having their lives turned upside down because of it. So what can we do?

It's possible to filter most fluorine from your drinking water. And you may be able to find ways to avoid paper products that contain Dupont fat barriers (staying away from fast foods is one way). But, despite what some detox product venders and "cleansing" advocates claim in the alternative medicine fields, you simply may not be able to get certain chemical residues out of your system using natural approaches (although it is possible to remove some heavy metals such as mercury by introducing natural chelating agents like cilantro or chlorella that bind with the metals). If your liver cannot recognize chemicals or molecular residues as toxins and selectively filter them out, how in the world are you going to get rid of them if natural chelation techniques don't work?

Our only option at the moment may be medical intervention via drug chelation therapies—that is if Big Pharma deems such therapies to be profitable in the long term. But Big Pharma probably won't push too hard for such therapies because it prefers to serve perpetually sick people by masking symptoms and having the profits continue to pour in. In any case, the science for removing such man-made chemicals—whether through herbal or drug means—just isn't well developed yet. So we must make due as wellness practitioners.

Yes, you will surely run across many alternative "detox protocols" and claims that seem to hold promise, but few will be well researched. Most will be personality-driven and/or designed to get you to open your wallet. Nonetheless, you should keep an open mind because wellness practice and closed minds do not work so well together. Consult your wellness professional if you are not sure how to evaluate such protocols.

How Toxins Affect Your Body

There are a plethora of signs and symptoms that can result from toxins hanging around in your system, or from your homeostatic balance not being optimal because of a poor diet and such. Problems include digestive issues, esophageal reflux, upset stomach, bloating and gas, diarrhea and constipation, low energy, PMS, headaches, irritability, skin rashes and conditions, chronic aches and pains, high cholesterol, food intolerances, alcohol intolerance, arthritic symptoms, weight gain, hormonal imbalance, and more. Of course, any of these signs and symptoms may have nothing to do with toxin accumulation in the direct sense and more to do with poor homeostasis, too much stress buildup, or even disease, but you must be ready to think about detoxification as part of your optimum wellness lifestyle. Most people need to.

Role of the Liver, GI tract, and Kidneys in Detoxification

Simply put, your liver is a vital and necessary part of your health. The liver's job is to detoxify your blood. All of the blood in your body runs through the liver, where it is cleansed.

The liver is like an air conditioning filter. If you haven't changed your AC filter lately, you will notice that it is dirty with a lot of dust and lint stuck to it. If you don't clean or change the filter regularly, your AC unit will become dirty, inefficient, and possibly even break down from the stress. Your liver is no different. It filters and detoxifies the blood. If you don't keep it "clean" and functioning normally, it begins to break down and your body suffers due to toxin accumulation.

The liver has two detoxification phases. In Phase 1, a toxin is altered into a less harmful, intermediate metabolic product. However, undesirable free radicals form during this phase. Your body must supply an adequate amount of anti-oxidants to neutralize the free radicals. This rids the body of unnecessary toxic interactions. But without a properly functioning liver or an adequate supply of anti-oxidants, liver cells can be damaged from the presence of the free radicals.

In Phase 2 of the detoxification process, a substance is added to the less harmful, intermediate product to form a water-soluble substance that can be moved out of the body via the colon or the kidneys. The result is an end of the toxic interaction and a cleansing of the body. For this phase to work, the liver, gastrointestinal tract, kidneys, and other excretory systems all have to be functioning well.

The gastro-intestinal (GI) tract works in conjunction with the liver in the detoxification system by providing a direct portal of exit for unwanted waste. The problem today is that the average American has a dysfunctional GI tract. From improper digestion to improper absorption of nutrients to improper elimination of waste, GI problems are pandemic. Acid-reducing medications such as the "Purple Pill™" are advertised to "relieve" problems associated with upset stomach and heartburn. The problem is that the stomach requires acid to digest food properly. By taking these meds, digestion is greatly hampered if not halted. Improper digestion leads to improper nutrition and consequently lower-bowel problems including constipation, irritable bowel syndrome, ulcers, and in extreme cases cancer of the colon. You can follow easy, basic steps to avoid these pitfalls and the need for such medications. The right steps can also ensure proper GI function and detoxification.

The kidneys further aid in detoxification by filtering out toxins and waste from the blood and eliminating them from the body through the urine. Simply drinking the right amount of water and avoiding the types of drinks that slowly and surely destroy health can help the kidneys work efficiently and effectively.

Benefits of Detoxification

A properly executed detoxification protocol includes:

- Restoring more normal detoxification processes and functions
- Eliminating free radical damage that speeds up the aging process
- Strengthening the immune system
- Improving overall health and organ function
- Eliminating old, unhealthy, detrimental habits, and substituting new, restorative, health-building habits so you can reclaim your health, your youth, your life!

The detox process should be safe, simple, comfortable, and rewarding. Not all detoxification programs are effective, safe, or even based on decent evidence. Much comes from myth and is fear-based. Some comes from sleight-of-hand that leads you to believe toxins and other nasty looking stuff is being extracted from your body. The Internet and infomercials are chock full of opportunities to lighten your wallet if you decide to hop onto the pseudo-detoxification bandwagon.

Constipation is one such area. For example, you're probably much better off changing your diet to eliminate constipation than using herbal detox products that are primarily laxatives. After all, taking laxatives will not cure constipation, and could easily make it worse. That's no better than the medical approach of masking symptoms!

Be wary of poorly researched or scam detox techniques like colonics or toxin-absorbing footpads. Also, footbaths that claim to "draw toxins" out of your feet into the water, thus changing its color, are frauds. The water color has nothing to do with toxins being drawn from the feet!

Nonetheless, authentic ionic footbath devices do stimulate your feet with negative ions that neutralize—through osmosis—excess free radicals in your blood and tissues. This allows your already burdened liver to more easily convert and then release toxic substances through sweat, urine, and so on (see Detox points #1 and #3 starting on page 207).

213

Also, avoid long-term fasting techniques like the "Master Cleanse," a 10-day detox plan that consists of nothing but lemon juice, maple syrup, and cayenne pepper. Fasting was all the rage about 20 or 30 years ago, but today we know that your body actually *needs* specific nutrients to aid its natural detoxification process. Heavy fasting doesn't supply those nutrients. Nonetheless, short-term elimination fasts can identify the source of food intolerances and allergies, especially if the fasts are professionally supervised or mentored.

When is it Best to Detox?

In 2008 outside Los Angeles, a three-day think-tank was set up involving some of the top experts in autism detoxification. By consensus, that group came up with the following *priority list* for achieving optimal health:

1. Healthy Living
2. Avoiding Electromagnetic Fields (EMF)
3. Clean Water
4. Healthy Food
5. Healthy Movement
6. Emotions & Relationships
7. Tests
8. Organ Support
9. Supplements
10. Detox Tools

Note that detoxification tools are on the list, *but at number 10.* Nine other factors come before it to help build health and provide support. Unfortunately, many self-diagnosing sick people consider detoxing, *first,* when they're not feeling well. But if you fail to follow an orderly process and instead begin detoxification prematurely or incorrectly, it can deteriorate your health even further and make you sicker than you already are.

Unless you are under the care of a wellness doctor who determines that your detoxification must be raised in priority before you can make any headway (which is true of many people), *you should avoid starting any toxin-removal regimen while you are sick.* You need to establish a healthy lifestyle and dietary habits <u>first</u>, so that you have a reserve that your body can draw on to allow your liver to do its job properly. Fail to do this and you can easily overwhelm your liver's ability to process the toxic substances being eliminated and you will become even sicker, wishing you had never done the detox in the first place. Please use caution and evaluate your current state of health before embarking on any kind of detoxification program. Allow your 5% (or more) professional care to weigh in!

Here's an important point to help you stay on center. It doesn't pay to get yourself all stressed out about the negative conditions present in our modern, chemical-laden world. That would just be jumping from the frying pan into the fire because emotional stress can endanger your health even more than lingering chemical toxins. Yes, do take reasonable actions to avoid toxins or cleanse your body of them, but it would be foolish to think you can get them all out using what we know at the moment. A reasonable approach can definitely help you counteract some of the onslaught of "damage by chemistry." But then go on and live your life. Life is meant to be lived, not feared. If you have been practicing maximum wellness, any toxin buildup will not have as much of an impact on you as someone who abuses his or her health through ignorance or lack of discipline.

Finally, if you're just starting out with your wellness practice, work with a professional who has a good reputation for safe, effective, comfortable detoxification protocols and who is willing to tell you how and why they work and show you the research. I've now given you enough background to ask some good questions!

The Ever-Expanding Role of Innate Intelligence

With respect to detoxification, keep in mind the growing scientific evidence that your body's innate intelligence can do more than you believe—much more in fact. Here's why.

Quantum physics has turned cause/effect on its head. Day by day it is teaching us that our consciousness—that which we consent to or believe to be true (openly or at the subconscious level)—limits the ways our innate intelligence can work to protect us and keep us healthy. This is similar to how cell receptors decide what can and can't enter our cells. If we are able to change our consciousness, then we are able to change our health and

how our genes express themselves. Big gains are possible here for those who are spiritually adventurous.

That is why the practice of wellness continues to expand for us. There is so much more we can learn. And that is also why the spiritual component of wellness plays such a large role in the physical, emotional, and mental areas of our lives.

* * *

In the previous chapter, I promised to talk more about choosing a wellness doctor, even if that doctor isn't a chiropractor. I'll now talk about that in some detail because it's important to you.

How Do You Find a Compatible Wellness Doctor?

So just how do you find wellness professionals—both chiropractors and others? How do you gage their qualifications, especially since "wellness" is still such a buzzword? After all, it's not always easy to figure out what a doctor's advertising means. In fact, the doctors themselves might not even be able to tell you what wellness means if pressed (see page 15 as a reminder). So let's dig more deeply into the doctor search because it's a common situation.

If you don't have access to a qualified wellness chiropractor in your area, you might try another type of doctor who is ready, willing, and able to enthusiastically support you in achieving your wellness goals as you now understand them. Are there good wellness doctors who are not chiropractors? Sure. Lots of them. They are usually considered "alternative" practitioners these days. Many are fine M.D.s and D.O.s who have carefully fit themselves into wellness practice. That is not always so easy for them to do because much of today's "healthcare" is dominated by pharmaceuticals and their self-interested advocates. Of course, that's changing, and rapidly. But maybe not rapidly enough.

Some alternative doctors are called naturopathic doctors or naturopathic medical doctors (NDs or NMDs). Naturopathic doctors teach their patients to use diet, exercise, lifestyle changes, and cutting-edge natural therapies to enhance their abilities to ward off and combat disease.

To start with, you would be unwise to choose a wellness practitioner simply because he or she is the closest or the cheapest. Instead, get a

216

recommendation from a local health food store or from a friend or relative who shares your goals for health.

Another option is to visit the website of the American Association of Naturopathic Physicians at www.naturopathic.org. You might find a good ND or NMD in your area if there are no practicing wellness DC's.

One more option is to look on the Internet for practitioners of complementary and alternative medicine (CAM). Still another is to visit www.ACAMnet.org to find doctors of all stripes who practice integrative or holistic medicine. That site hosts the American College for Advancement in Medicine (ACAM). Some of those practitioners *could* be right for you although most won't. You will need to read about their practice specialties and perhaps interview them to see where they really stand. You might even have to try them out for a while to see if they practice the kind of wellness that supports your *Reclaim 24* lifestyle.

However, I want to be clear about this point: **It will be unproductive to work with a wellness doctor who does not advocate maintaining spinal health throughout the year as a preventative measure for maintaining good nervous system function. Waiting for symptoms to arise is too late.** *That is not wellness practice.*

As you know by now, a malfunctioning nervous system will not get you where you want to go with wellness. This means your doctor should be happy to recommend a good chiropractor to help you maintain a healthy spine through regular attention. If he or she is hesitant about that, start looking elsewhere. The doctor is asking you to practice wellness with one arm tied behind your back. Here's the crux of the matter:

> **Not many people will regularly visit a doctor when they are already feeling great. Yet, a growing number of us who want to be and do our best are visiting wellness doctors regularly. A yearly "physical" is not enough.**

Indeed, the yearly physical common under the allopathic healthcare model is not preventative. That model screens for the early onset of disease. That's fine if the screening doesn't create its own problems, but disease screening is not a substitute for wellness care. It's an adjunct.

Once you are closing in on or even "trying out" a prospective practitioner, look for the following conditions or behaviors to help you evaluate what kind of wellness practice your doctor is running. And don't expect perfection! It's hard to come by. You may have to augment your approach, perhaps even using several complementary health professionals, to make things work for you. Once you become proficient in wellness practice, developing your "support team" will be easier for you.

Education and Inspiration. Your practitioner should provide inspiration, encouragement, and advice that empower *you* to take charge of your health and adopt a wellness lifestyle. After all, it is your body that does the healing and not the doctor. In the best of all worlds, he or she will offer lifestyle education and counseling programs. A good wellness doctor won't be afraid to "transfer" elements of wellness care to you as you become more adept at handling it. He or she will want to see you spread your wings!

Holistic Approach. Is this doctor looking at all aspects of health and wellness, and looking at the body as a whole rather than just some parts, chemicals, or functions in isolation? For example, viewing your wellness efforts from the perspective of the five pillars of optimized health is a holistic approach. In truth, all of the cells in your body need to be functioning at their best if you are to experience maximum wellness.

An Ongoing, Tailored Plan of Prevention. The practitioner offers an ongoing wellness-care plan and approach, tailored to you, that does not just have you returning when something is wrong. Yes, the doctor periodically screens, but the screening looks for optimum function more than pathologies. The intention is to restore a healthful function to the nervous system, organs, glands, and body structure—with your help. When your body is functioning healthfully, pathologies seldom arise. Not only that, you should be able to recognize your own progress and not just take the doctor's word for it.

Function, Not Feeling. Is your doctor assessing your health based on how you are feeling or how you are functioning? Yes, your doctor should be trying to relieve any symptoms of discomfort that you might have, but true wellness care means ensuring that your body is functioning as well as it can at all times, not waiting for symptoms to tell you that something is seriously wrong. Also, is the doctor using techniques and advice with which you are comfortable? You need to ask yourself the questions, "Are this doctor's techniques designed to improve my function and wellness, or merely dull symptoms I might be experiencing? Are the techniques proven and safe?"

Doesn't Constrain His/Her Approach to Qualify for Insurance Benefits. The practitioner doesn't base the frequency, duration, and type of your treatment on whether your insurance covers it. Remember, insurance programs are the product of an allopathic healthcare model. They are still years away from being wellness oriented.

Do You "Click?" It's a hard thing to define, but if you intend to work with a doctor who is going to help you practice wellness for the rest of your life (or the rest of his/hers), it's important that you "connect" with that individual. You should feel comfortable enough to ask all the tough questions you need to ask to understand your wellness level and to expand your knowledge of self-care. *Above all, your doctor should be a good listener.* No one knows more about your body than you do. Your doctor must listen to you and be "present" to absorb what you are saying, and even be flexible enough to change direction if your needs are not being met.

Does the Doctor Look and Act Healthy? Appearance tells you a lot! The best person to guide you towards health and wellness is someone who has "been there and done that." He or she knows the road you need to take and has probably made plenty of mistakes so you don't have to.

Qualifications? Be sure that the doctor is adequately qualified in his or her practice area. A doctor should also have sufficient training to advise you on the areas of wellness that are important to you—or be prepared to refer you to someone who does. Choose only licensed practitioners. There is more protection to that than meets the eye.

How Much Does It Cost? You should be informed of the fees and charges up front and in an open and honest way. Be sure that the fees for the care you require agree with what you are prepared to invest for your health. With this said, by now I hope you view wellness support as an investment and not an expense. What is your health worth?

* * *

Once you find a compatible wellness doctor or team of doctors, please don't leave your children, spouse, or parents home to get sick while you are getting wellness care, counseling, and generally healthy. Make wellness practice a family affair! All of you will be happier and healthier for it.

But What If You're in An Emergency Situation?

If you are acutely ill or suffering from an emergency or accident of some sort, then you might need more than wellness care. In fact, you might need some high-level emergency medical care to get you through the situation. This may or may not require a different practitioner. Even if you are under emergency care, though, you will still want someone to help you address the underlying causes of your general problems so you can improve your state of wellness for the long term. That helps you avoid more crises or even emergencies down the road!

My Wellness Center Practice

Here I'll describe my personal practice philosophy and approach to give you additional ideas about what you might look for in a wellness practitioner who also supports your self-care interests. You'll find that different practitioners focus on different factors that complement their unique backgrounds, understandings, and interests. That's fine.

For instance, I support my patients along the lines of the five pillars of optimized health that I've talked about at length in this book and which are the foundation for *Reclaim 24*. Others might not focus in the same way. You just need to know that *your* practitioner can support you the way you need and want to be supported. After all, if you've started practicing a *Reclaim 24* lifestyle, you no longer dwell in the myth and ignorance that lead to so many bad choices and eventually the Conveyor Belt to a Living Hell. For you, the smoke is clearing!

Many people who end up at a wellness doctor's office for the first time have symptoms of some sort. Not you, of course. Your first visit to my wellness center would be to embark upon or to expand your wellness program, right?

Well, we can hope.

In truth, the vast majority of people who come to my center are indeed looking to embark on a wellness program because they know I have a reputation as a wellness expert. Some of my patients even affectionately call me "Dr. Wellness." I like that! On the other hand, most of the new arrivals also show up with symptoms, and often pain. Daily stress, injuries, and a lifetime of poor choices certainly take their toll. Pain has a way of inspiring some people to change habits!

You should know that today's wellness chiropractors are not just therapy-oriented back-and-neck doctors. Wellness chiropractors focus on programs and approaches that support "optimized living." However, many chiropractors limit their practices to traditional therapeutic support and short-term pain relief—typically in the neck, back, and shoulders. There's certainly nothing wrong with such doctors. They don't use drugs, and they'll typically give you quick relief.

What's more, countless numbers of people simply don't subscribe to a self-care lifestyle that wellness doctors might promote. They just don't have the self-discipline, knowledge, or trust in themselves to take personal responsibility for their health. A large part of this stems from having accepted a medical model that has coaxed them into becoming lifelong "medical dependents." They happily subordinate themselves to medical authorities because they don't feel they have any option. Such people prefer to pay M.D.s to remove their discomforts when they arise. Self-care is not much of a consideration. As you can tell, I'm biased about this medical dependency, but for good reason.

Most often, those who settle for quick relief just return home to continue with the same, poor lifestyle choices that brought on their pain or other problems in the first place. With time, their pain-relief visits become more frequent while their overall health continues to decline. They make their choices and they pay accordingly. However, many people today are taking more of a wellness or alternative-care route because traditional health care continues to disappoint.

Like most healing professionals, I don't feel it's okay to have pain or depleted health. Though I'm a wellness-oriented practitioner, I always look to relieve distress symptoms for someone who initially comes to me seeking relief. In some cases I'll even refer such a person to medical or other professionals when I think that's called for. Many times it is! Any health practitioner who thinks he or she has all the answers or all the comprehensive professional skills to support your health needs is, well, downright dangerous (in my opinion).

Okay, wellness chiropractors can also help you get quick relief when necessary. Yet, there's so much more you can have if you decide to *practice* wellness through the lifestyle habits you choose—those habits under your control. In other words, the use of wellness chiropractic becomes just one of many positive lifestyle habits. It complements all the other proactive things you do to achieve and maintain the greatest state of well-being that you can.

221

Services & Approaches I Emphasize at My Wellness Center

If you came to my center to get help with your wellness quest, I'd tell you that I see myself as a wellness mentor and healing assistant ready and willing to help you thrive in conjunction with your body's natural ability to heal itself. I'd also tell you that most of my regular patients[43] devote considerable effort towards developing new habits that build wellness. After all, they want the most mileage from their God-given potentials. And I wouldn't hesitate to tell you that I much prefer to work with people like that! They inspire me to be my best and give my best.

Of course, I would emphasize the five pillars of optimized health, and you would see charts on the wall to that effect. At the bottom of it all, I'd tell you *why* I focus on those five pillars. It's because:

1. I want you to enjoy the healing benefits of an unblocked nervous system.
2. I want you to see how you can stop creating your own health problems.
3. I want you to see through the myths that rob you of any chance of experiencing optimized living.
4. I want you to experience the benefits that come from wellness practice and responsible self-care.

If you came to my center with pain symptoms, I'd surely want to know what your immediate goals are and what your lifestyle is like. I'd want to know if you are willing to change some habits, or whether you've simply come for a pain-relieving adjustment and a pat on the shoulder. I'd tell you I can probably relieve your symptoms in short order, but also that it will seldom be your best answer for achieving long-term health and wellness. Yet, short-term relief sure beats living with pain!

I'd explain that, with my wellness approach, I help a patient correct spinal stress or damage, but that I also look for *causes* of stress or

---

[43] I continue to use the socially accepted word, "patient," with some hesitation. The term carries medical baggage and implies a dependency or even subordinate relationship. "Partner-in-wellness" would be a better description for an enlightened patient who advocates wellness, self-care, and self-responsibility for making choices. But such a phrase still sounds awkward, so I'll stick with the familiar "patient" until our culture warms up to something more descriptive!

damage. In the process, I would make the following point crystal clear because sometimes distress symptoms clear up with just a few sessions of TLC:

> **A lack of distress symptoms does not equal wellness! Wellness has more to do with how your body is *supposed to work* than how you feel at any one moment of time.**

I would try ever so hard to drive that point home because the public is hypnotized in the **medical mindset** of assuming one is healthy once symptoms are gone and test numbers look okay (all of which can be misleading or simply wrong). For example, a large number of my patients are middle-aged women who have been told they have thyroid insufficiency and have been taking various trade-name medications (usually Synthroid™) to get their laboratory thyroid numbers back into the "normal" range. But they still feel lousy, and with good reason. The *vast* majority of these women have Hashimoto's disease, an autoimmune condition that attacks thyroids and makes them malfunction. Dosing with the synthetic hormone, Synthroid, to make the lab numbers look good *will not* control Hashimoto's and the thyroid gland will simply continue to deteriorate. Meanwhile, the lousy feelings will often be misdiagnosed as depression, cyclothymia, PMS, chronic fatigue syndrome, fibromyalgia, or anxiety disorder.

Seeking only symptom relief means deeper causes of problems are being overlooked. Unchecked, the problems hang around behind the scenes to do their dirty deeds again and again in the future, sometimes even wearing different disguises (symptoms). Then, back to the doctor for more, quick symptom removal. But here's the thing: *Just as sickness development is a process, healing is also a process—not just an event marked by a quick fix.*

All other things being equal, the less long-term damage you exhibit, the faster you heal. Of course, as a wellness doctor, I don't prescribe drugs to mask symptoms. I use methods that help patients heal without them having to resort to the insult of drugs or surgery. Some in the medical field are not happy with the chiropractic or wellness approach, but when their "healthcare" statistics and malpractice insurance premiums[44]

---

[44] Mal-practice insurance for a chiropractor is as little as what you pay for a year of auto insurance. Many M.D.'s pay $200,000 or more per year for malpractice

are revealed, they don't have too much to crow about. Professional chiropractic is truly safe as well as effective. But beware the homegrown back-and-neck cracker.

I would also explain that once the acute phase of your care has done its job, falling back to regular care helps you dwell at a higher level on your personal wellness scale—which you now know has little to do with lack of symptoms. I would further offer you a choice as to the recovery or wellness level you want to achieve with your visits, and I would point out the likely implications of making choices among

> *"The person who takes medicine must recover twice, once from the disease, and once from the medicine." – William Usler, M.D.*

the options you have available. Some people want a Rolls Royce. Others are happy with a Honda Civic. It's a matter of temperament and priorities. Less frequently, pocketbook. Not everyone is ready or willing to shoot for maximum wellness, but many are willing to go beyond being a drug buyer and tester (guinea pig) for Big Pharma.

In your first two visits, I would be taking a personal history, obtaining a metabolic profile, and scheduling diagnostic tests. These tests might include x-rays (I'd be a fool to adjust your neck or spine without them), a G.I. panel, an orthopedic and neurological exam, a comprehensive blood panel, and a hormone and neurotransmitter evaluation. Your first two visits, along with the proper diagnostic lab work, would tell me everything I would need to know to assess your health situation and offer a wellness care plan that would work best for you (unless I think you need to see another doctor instead).

Remember, it wouldn't be my job to mask your symptoms with drugs and then send you off after one or two visits. That's what medicine does. And you wouldn't be "well" just because your symptoms passed. It would be my job to dig deeper for the cause(es) of your distress symptoms. Once found, I could help you in better ways than just to alleviate symptoms.

* * *

Chapter 15 made it clear that there's a giant leap from disease care to health care. It involves shattering the fiction that prevents maximum

---

insurance. If anyone knows about risk and safety, it's insurance companies. That's how they stay in business.

wellness—and there's plenty of fiction going around. And what is the greatest part of that fiction? It is the belief that the allopathic model of healthcare really is "healthcare."

The allopathic model, *as a healthcare system,* casts a long, dark, cold shadow behind it, leaving all in its shadow shivering from the lack of life-giving sun. Even many fine M.D.s, deeply committed to serving their patients, shiver from the cold of drug protocols forced on them by Big Pharma; from the stern control of a medical hierarchy influenced by Big Pharma; and from ever-tightening control of government regulators influenced by—you guessed it—Big Pharma. Good doctors can risk their professional reputations and careers—and possibly even their licenses and freedom to dwell among us—if they endeavor to serve their patients from a wellness perspective instead of from the authoritarian stranglehold of conventional medicine. Straying from conventional practice is not welcome unless the power elite first gives its blessings. M.D.s who practice wellness must be careful how they go about it.

The good news is that there is sun and warmth out there for you if you're willing to step out of the shadows. But it's not until you're willing to take that step of your own accord that your God-given potential to experience maximum wellness is revealed to you. Until then, it's a secret.

As a quick summary, in the best of all worlds, to practice maximum wellness is to:

1. Embrace your many self-care opportunities in the four crucial categories of wellness behaviors described starting on page 25, and

2. Partner with a wellness doctor, or a team of wellness profession-als as the case may be, to help you navigate the five key areas where you might need some professional support.
   a) Nervous System (structural perspective)
   b) Organs and Glands (hormonal perspective)
   c) Detoxification
   d) Nutrition
   e) Fitness/Motion/Exercise

Getting Your Wellness Education

I'm a knowledge addict, and I suggest you become one, too, if possible. I love to share what I know with others so they can reach their optimum levels of wellness—levels that support optimized living. I read all the latest research and information about how to be incredibly healthy, and I've continued my formal education with advanced training in neurology, fitness, nutrition, and anti-aging. I also hold certifications in spinal trauma and functional endocrinology.

Because of what I've learned, I urge you to be proactive about your health and your family's health. In this book I've given you as many ways as are reasonable within a limited number of pages to learn how to get healthy and stay healthy without the continuous onslaught of drugs and surgery. The more you know, the healthier you can become—BUT ONLY IF YOU ACT ON YOUR KNOWLEDGE.

So, yes, continue to expand your knowledge about wellness, but don't stop with knowledge, alone, or you'll just get intellectual constipation and become a consummate bore to everyone around you. Start practicing the wellness lifestyle behaviors as discussed in Chapter 3, even if you are still wet behind the ears in overall wellness knowledge!

The Effect of Wellness on Your Pocketbook

Your proactive wellness program helps save you a lot of money and heartache over time. On the surface, you might ask yourself why you should visit a doctor when you're feeling good. And maybe you question the value of organic or other high-quality foods, and possibly nutritional products intended to keep you functioning at a high level on the wellness scale. All that stuff costs more than what people typically spend, right?

Well, yes, but what people are you thinking about? Especially as they get into their later years? Do you know what drug prescriptions cost these days? Medical care? *Not having* medical care insurance? Even *having* medical care insurance?

Here's something to think about. The journal, *Health Affairs,* reported early in 2005 that soaring medical bills cause half of all U.S. bankruptcies. Moreover, most people sent into debt by illness are middle-class workers with health insurance!

Look, I'm not going to cover the financial value of wellness in this book. You can easily get an eye-opening picture for yourself by going to google.com on the Internet, for example. Enter the search phrase, **do wellness programs pay for themselves**. Reading summaries of what's been learned will keep you busy for the better part of a day. I just want to point out that, when all the factors are considered, your personal wellness program is likely to cost much less than being financially enslaved by the pharmaceutical industry and the false hopes of surgery and drug-induced solutions to health problems.

And don't be taken in by the health insurance argument without some careful evaluation. Health insurance isn't working for people as it used to. In fact, it's starting to look less and less like true "insurance" and more and more like an expensive talisman against illness.

At the heart of it all, the value of wellness, first and foremost is … being well. Truly well! How much value do you put on that? What's it worth to you to be well? What's it worth to you to experience the vitality that life offers those who have the gumption to step out of the cold? What chances do you think you have of being well under the umbrella of drugs and surgery that treat degenerative diseases, *especially if the diseases aren't necessary?* And last, what's it worth to you not to spend 10, 20, or even more years on the Conveyor Belt to a Living Hell? 'Nuff said.

The Wellness Lifestyle

The wellness lifestyle recognizes a crucial fact that differentiates health care from sick care: **True health is about how our bodies work, not about how we feel.** For example, if you become nauseous when you ingest things harmful to you, then your body is working just fine. But you're not feeling so hot. Suppress the nausea with a drug and you'll feel better. Suppress it long enough and you might not be feeling anything at all!

As children, we learned to think of sickness as having obvious symptoms, but this belief is killing us as adults. These days, huge numbers of people are dropping dead from lifestyle-induced diseases whose first symptoms are often … well … death! True health is optimum physical, mental, emotional, and spiritual well-being and not merely the absence of disease or infirmity.

Drinking more clean water; eating nutritious foods; getting regular exercise; reducing physical, environmental, emotional, and mental stress; and engaging in virtually every other healthy habit that we know about so far produces larger dividends when combined with a properly working nervous system. That's why a wellness center such as mine specializes in helping patients gain true health by getting their bodies and higher components of their being to function at their best.

227

The Inescapable Role You Play

Please understand that a wellness doctor can't do *everything* for you. Not even close, in fact. For example:

❑ If you're not getting the right nutrition, the bright flame of your self-healing forces will dwindle to a flicker. That flicker may not be sufficient to handle the stress loads you have on your body, mind, and emotions. A wellness doctor can't change your eating habits.

❑ If you're not getting the *right type* of regular exercise that you need both to regulate your metabolism and to flex your spine the way it wants to be flexed in order to power your brain and keep your nervous system stimulated, then your health and appearance will just continue to decline. Professional wellness care can't alter poor choices or lack of motivation for maintaining fitness.

❑ If you choose to dwell in a "caustic" environment of poor friends and associates and you're not taking reasonable precautions to avoid toxins in the air you breathe, the water you use, and the food you eat, your choices will weigh heavily on your ability to achieve maximum wellness. All these additional environmental stressors may easily overload your healing responses, even if you visit wellness doctors regularly.

❑ If you choose to dwell in noxious thoughts and feelings, there is no way to achieve maximum wellness.

❑ If you're not nurturing yourself spiritually, everything becomes harder for you and those around you. That's just the way it is.

The point is that maximum wellness falls 95% into your hands through right education and right action. Wellness is 95% self-care!

Got Passion? Then Get on the Fast Track!

Even though regular wellness care provided by professionals creates a solid foundation for optimized living, you can use parts I and II of this book to engage in a self-care, fitness, and nutrition program that takes you much further. That is, assuming you have the self-motivation. Some wellness doctors are able to formally help you with such efforts. There's no reason you can't sculpt your body into a shape you are much prouder

228

of, and gain extra vitality to boot. So, if the reflection you see in the mirror isn't the one you want to look at, take the initiative to change it! Others will help you professionally if you need it. And everyone around you will be happy you did.

To summarize the comprehensive benefits present in this book, benefits that amount to my unique blueprint for a *Reclaim 24* lifestyle:

- ❏ I've told you what wellness and wellness practice *really* are so you can immediately recognize them, work with them, and choose professionals to help you achieve your goals.

- ❏ I've shown you how aging primarily comes from stress buildup and not from the parade of calendar years. I've also shown you how to reduce the different types of stress that spoil your life.

- ❏ I've shown you how you can enjoy better moods for yourself and those around you.

- ❏ I've discussed how the subconscious mind works so you can more easily overcome the failure habit and the negative influences of others who would have you fail.

- ❏ I've shown you ways to replace harmful habits with good ones.

- ❏ I've shown you how to reshape your body into something you can be proud of.

- ❏ I've shown you how to choose foods for health and wellness without turning your life upside down. Also, how to increase your energy supply so you can live life with more vitality.

- ❏ I've given you an approach that you can use to prove to yourself within 12 weeks or less that you're on the right track with your maximum wellness program, fitness, and appearance.

- ❏ I've given you a quick overview of copious research that shows why the practice of medicine, although crucial for crisis care, cannot support you in your *wellness* efforts.

- ❏ I've told you what you need to know to start recognizing the large gap between having no symptoms of illness and living in a state of true wellness. Also, how to bridge that gap.

- ❏ I've chipped away at the key myths and illusions that rob you of your quality of life.

- ❏ I've talked about the healing and vitalizing benefits of an unblocked nervous system, along with the prolonged youth that come with them—benefits for the entire family.

- ❏ I've discussed innate intelligence and how it is forever working in the background to support your efforts; even changing the ways your genes express themselves!

- ❏ I've given you the tools of wellness practice that allow you to slow your aging process to a crawl so that you can extend the vitality of your 20's and 30's for many decades. This includes an understanding of how hormones affect wellness.

- ❏ Finally, I've given you every reason to believe that you don't *have* to become a long-haul passenger on the Conveyor Belt to a Living Hell or resident of the Pits of Despair!

* * *

So there you have it! Follow my 12-week *Reclaim 24* Action Plan as fast-track proof that you can indeed change for the better, proof that you have golden opportunities to alter your life in ways that you thought had abandoned you.

Then embrace Part III of this book in order to soar!

Yes, death is inevitable, but many aspects of aging are reversible. Please remember this:

> **Health is the product of correct living. Early aging, sickness, and disease are the products of incorrect choices, bad information, and a faulty medical model.**

That's it, friend. I've shown you how to launch a lifestyle program that helps you stop creating your own health problems—a program that wants you to walk, always, with a bounce in your step and a gleam in your eye. Such is our God-given opportunity for a rich life. What will you do with your opportunity?

www.drcharleswebb.com

Appendix A:
Reclaim 24 Workout Illustrations

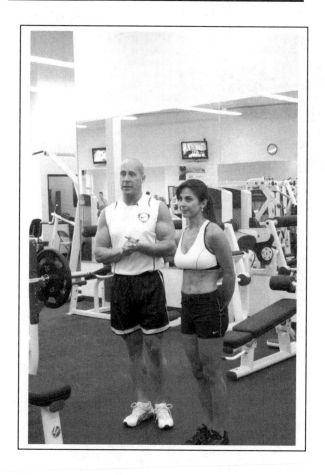

Dr. Webb and fitness associate, Michelle Heguy,
planning *Reclaim 24* photo shoot.

Chest: Upright Chest Press

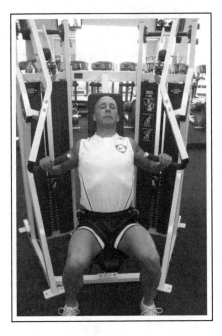

Starting and Finishing Position

Adjust the seat height on the chest-press machine. When you are properly seated, the handles will be under tension. Slowly press the handles outward and hold the outward extension (midpoint position) for a one count. Your elbows will be near locking. Then slowly bring the handles back to your starting position. Repeat.

Midpoint Position

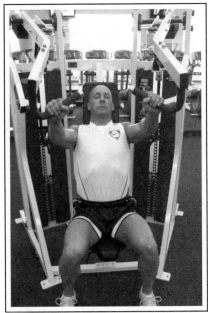

Chest: Flat Bench Flyes

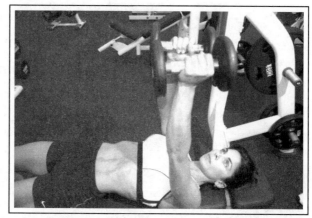

**Starting and
Finishing
Position**

Sit down on the edge of a bench with a dumbbell in each hand. Then lie back, keeping the dumbbells close to your chest and your feet flat on the floor. Then press the weights up, as shown, to start.

With your elbows slightly bent, slowly lower the dumbbells out to the sides to a point where they are even with the bench. Inhale as you lower. Then, after holding for a count of one, slowly raise them back to the starting position, exhaling on the way up.

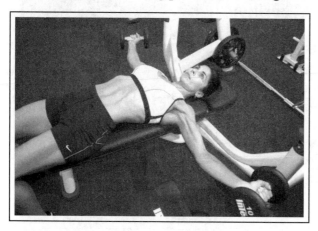

**Midpoint
Position**

233

Shoulders: Seated Dumbbell Press

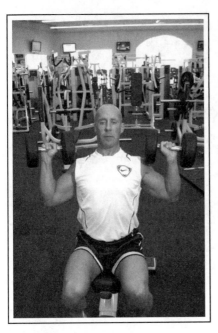

Starting and Finishing Position

Sit on the end of the bench with your feet flat on the floor. Hold a dumbbell in each hand at shoulder height. Keep your elbows out and your palms facing forward.

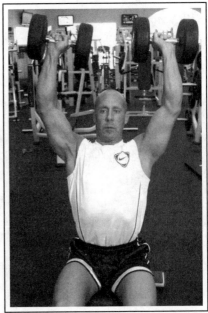

Midpoint Position

Press the dumbbells upward until your arms are nearly locked out, but not quite. Keep your palms facing forward. Allow the dumbbells to get close to each other at the top of the press. Then slowly lower the dumbbells to the starting position.

Shoulders: Standing Dumbbell Laterals

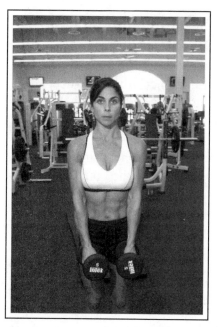

Starting and Finishing Position

Stand with your feet about shoulder width, your arms down, and your palms facing each other. Then, keeping your arms straight, raise them to each side. It's important to keep your palms facing downward as you raise the weights so that the exercise will work your shoulders rather than your biceps.

Midpoint Position

At the top of the lift, your arms *and your weights* will be parallel to the floor. Hold for a count of one and slowly lower to the starting position.

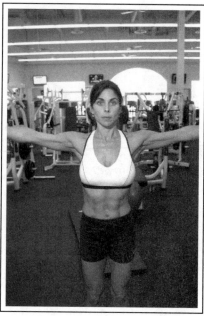

Back: Wide-Grip Pulldowns

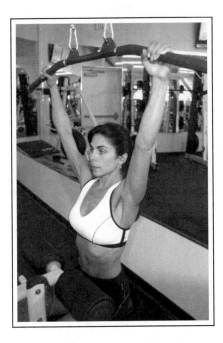

Starting and Finishing Position

First, check that the kneepads on the pulldown machine are adjusted so your thighs fit snugly under them while you are seated. Then, firmly grasp a *wide* bar on the machine so that your hands are separated by about twice your shoulder width (you'll need to stand to grab the bar). Then, holding onto the bar, seat yourself under the personally adjusted kneepads.

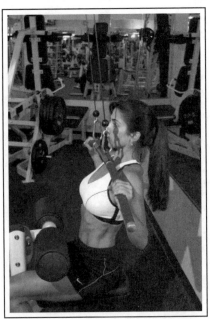

Midpoint Position

Slowly pull the bar down to the top of your chest or collarbone area, *but not lower*. Then slowly let the bar up to your starting position, which will still be under tension.

Back: One-Arm Dumbbell Rows

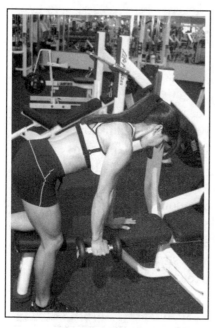

Starting and Finishing Position

Start with your right foot flat on the floor and your left knee resting on a flat bench. Then lean forward so you're supporting the weight of your upper body with your left arm on the bench. Your back should be almost parallel to the floor.

Reach down and pick up the dumbbell with your right hand. Look straight ahead instead of at the floor in order to keep your back straight.

Midpoint Position

Focus on pulling your elbow as far back as it can go. The dumbbell should end up roughly parallel to your torso. After you've lifted the weight as far as you can while still holding the rest of your body in the same position, slowly lower and repeat for the designated number of reps. Then repeat the whole exercise on your left side.

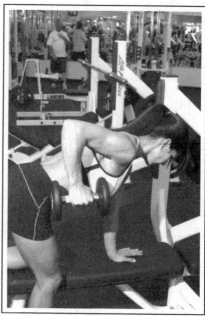

237

Triceps: Close-Grip Pushdowns

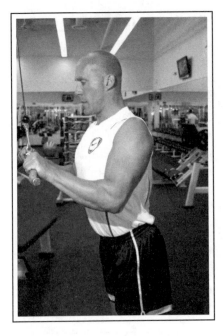

Starting and Finishing Position

This exercise is performed with a high-cable machine. Grip the bar with palms down and slightly narrower than shoulder width. Position your forearms so that they are nearly parallel to the ground to start. Keep your feet shoulder-width apart for added stability, and bend your knees slightly. Your wrists should be kept straight for the whole exercise. Tighten your abdominals to stabilize your upper torso and keep it from swaying.

Midpoint Position

Push the bar down and in toward your legs (a circular motion) until your arms are straight and your elbows locked. Keep your upper arms close to your body, and make those triceps flex at the bottom of the stroke for a count of one. Then slowly allow the bar to rise to the starting position for the next rep.

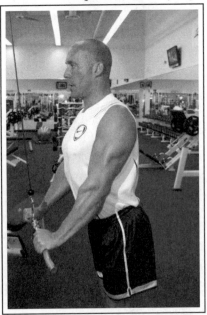

Triceps: Lying Triceps Press

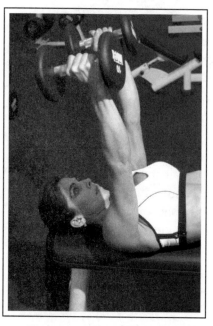

Starting and Finishing Position

Lie down on a flat bench with a dumbbell in each hand, arms extended over your head. You are looking straight up at the dumbbells. Your palms should be facing each other in this position and for the entire exercise.

Midpoint Position

Bend your elbows and *slowly* lower the dumbbells toward your shoulders, not toward your head. Your upper arms should remain stationary, perpendicular to the floor. *Don't let them tip backward.* That's cheating!

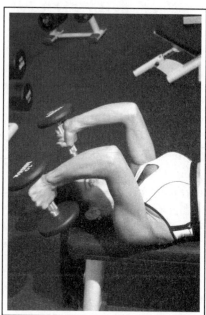

Biceps: Standing Dumbbell Curls

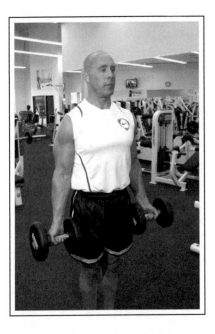

Starting and Finishing Position

Stand with your arms at your sides, with a dumbbell in each hand. Your focus should be on lifting the weights by flexing your biceps. You do not "swing" or change the position of *any* body part except your forearms, which curl upward.

Midpoint Position

With your palms initially facing forward, curl both arms, lifting the dumbbells slowly toward your shoulders. You want your biceps to do the work with your other muscles just keeping you in a stable position.

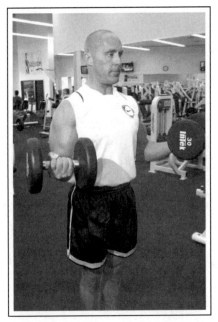

Biceps: Preacher Curls

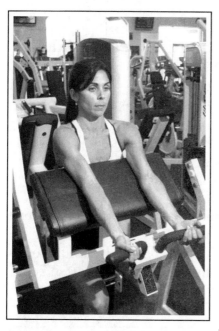

Starting and Finishing Position

Adjust the machine so the seat is comfortable and you can reach the handlebars easily. Set the weight for your current fitness level. Reach down and grasp the handle bar with an underhand grip, palms facing up. Press the back of your arms firmly against the arm pad and extend your elbows *without locking them.*

Midpoint Position

Tighten your abdominal muscles and straighten your back. Slowly lift the bar upward towards your chin until your arms reach your shoulders. Focus on contracting your bicep muscles at the top of the motion. Then slowly lower the bar back to your starting position, arms extended. Keep your elbows loose. Repeat for additional reps.

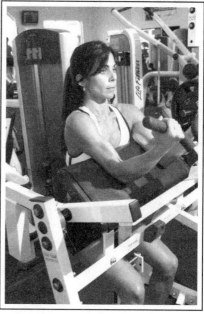

Quadriceps: Leg Extensions

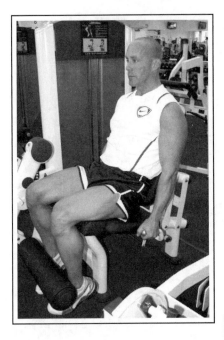

Starting and Finishing Position

Hook your ankles behind the roller pad of the leg-extension machine. The roller pad should be adjusted to rest on the lower part of your shins, *not* on the tops of your feet or in the middle of your shins. To keep your hips from lifting during the exercise, grasp the handles on the side of the machine to keep your bottom in place.

Midpoint Position

Straighten your legs, lifting the weight with your quads until your knees are straight. Always try for the fullest range of motion you can—all the way up, and all the way back down.

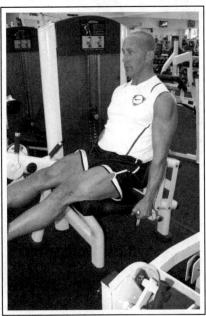

Quadriceps: Leg Press

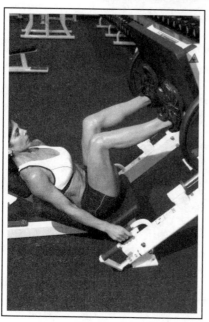

Starting and Finishing Position

On the leg-press machine, place your feet about shoulder width apart, toes slightly pointed out on the pressing platform. Hold the handles to keep your hips in place as you press the platform upward.

Midpoint Position

Slowly press the weight upward, being sure to push with your heels rather than your toes. And don't quite lock your knees at the top. Then slowly bring the platform back to its starting position for your next rep.

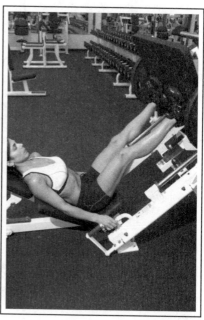

243

Hamstrings: Lying Leg Curls

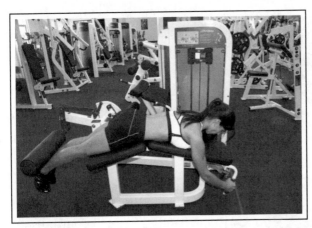

Starting and Finishing Position

Lie face-down on a lying-curl machine. Adjust your position so that the roller pad lies on the back of your ankles. In your starting position, the roller pad may already be under some tension.

Curl your legs up, and bring your feet as close to your hips as possible. Ideally, the roller pad (or pads) should touch the top of your hamstrings. Hold this fully contracted position for a count of one before *slowly* lowering the pad back to your starting position for the next rep.

Midpoint Position

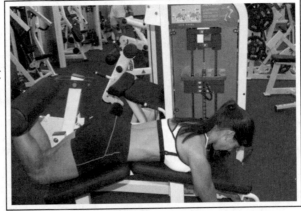

Hamstrings: Dumbbell Lunges

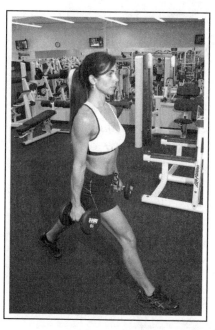

Step Position

In the starting position, stand erect with your feet together and the weights at your side with palms facing each other. The photo doesn't show the starting position. It shows the forward step taken with the right foot as the lunge movement begins.

Midpoint Position

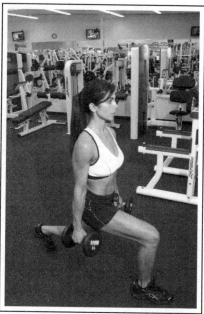

After stepping forward, bend at your knees and lower your hips until your left knee is just a few inches off the floor. Then push with your right leg, raising yourself back up to the starting point. Then repeat with your left leg. Throughout the exercise, don't lift your (forward) "lunge" foot. Keep it flat on the floor. You need to step far enough forward so that, at the full lunge position, your knee will be above your ankle and not in front of it.

245

Calves: Seated Calf Raises

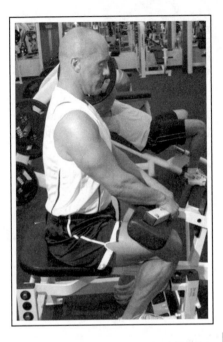

Starting and Finishing Position

Position yourself on a seated calf-raise machine with the balls of your feet on the platform and the kneepad on the lower part of your front thigh close to your knee. Keep your upper body still during the exercise, and focus on your calves.

Midpoint Position

Slowly raise your heels as your thighs press against the thigh pads. Flex hard and hold to a count of one. Then slowly lower your thigh so that your heels go as far below your toes as possible, thus stretching your calves to the maximum. Then repeat the next rep.

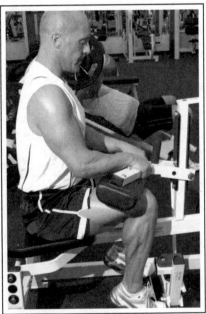

Calves: One-Legged Calf Raise

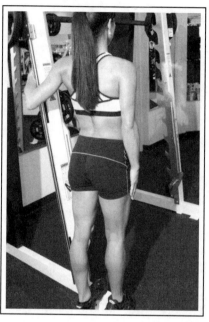

Starting and Finishing Position

Start with the ball of one foot resting on step or block so that your heel can be lowered far below the ball of your foot. You may also hold a dumbbell in the opposite hand to add more resistance to the exercise. Hold onto something for stability during the movement.

Midpoint Position

First, lower your heel below the ball of your foot as far as you can, thus stretching your calf to the maximum. Then press upward on your toe as far as possible, contracting your calf muscle. Hold that position for a count of one, and then repeat the movement for the required reps. Repeat the process for the other calf.

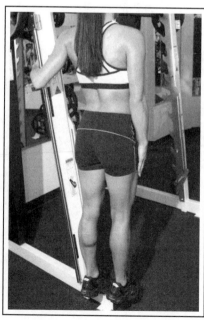

Abdominals: Pelvic Roll-Ups

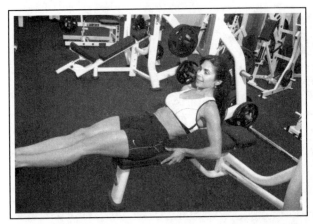

Starting and Finishing Position

Seated on the end of a flat bench, lay back with your legs extended and knees locked, propping up your torso with your hands (you don't want to start out from a totally flat position because that will place additional stress on your back and also use back muscles at the beginning of the movement rather than your abdominals.

Raise your knees toward your chest while simultaneously lifting your torso with your arms to end up in a "roll-up" position. Slowly return to the starting position and repeat.

Midpoint Position

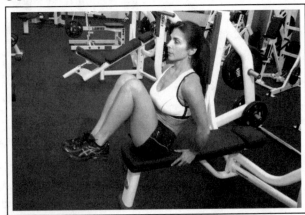

Abdominals: Twist Crunches

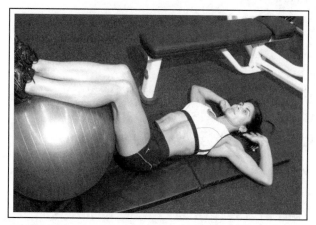

Starting and Finishing Position

Using an exercise ball to prop up your legs, place your hands behind your head so that your fingers are giving light support to your head as you raise your torso. *Do not lock your fingers together*. Then *smoothly* raise yourself and try to touch your left knee with your right elbow.

Hold your "crunched" position for a count of one. Then slowly lower yourself flat and repeat by touching your right knee with your left elbow. Alternate the left-right crunch as needed for your routine.

Beginning the Lift Before the Midpoint Position

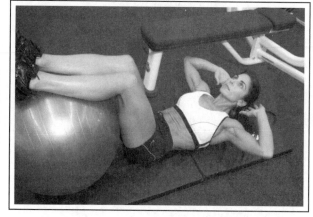

Every day my patients tell me—in one way or another—that my life's work and passion for wellness practice and wellness mentoring have been justified. Lives are changing! The success that these patients are having with *Reclaim 24* makes me leap out of bed in the morning. (Sometimes I can't even sleep at night because of the excitement, but that's another story.)

My patients are my walking, talking, breathing, "proof of concept" that the **Five Pillars of Optimized Health** at the foundation of *Reclaim 24* are right on target. For those patients, my program has been the gift that just keeps on giving. And that sure makes my day!

Appendix B:
Reclaim 24 Food Guide

Meat/Fish /Poultry	Serving Size	Calories	Protein (g)	Carbs (g)	Fat (g)
Top Sirloin	4 oz.	180	30	0	6
Top Round	4 oz.	190	36	0	4
Lean Ground Beef (85-90%)	4 oz.	263	28	0	16
Skinless Chicken Breast	4 oz.	165	31	0	4
Skinless Turkey Breast	4 oz.	135	30	0	1
Pork Tenderloin	4 oz.	164	28	0	5
Salmon	4 oz.	184	27	0	7
Halibut	4 oz.	140	27	0	3
Canned Light Tuna	4 oz.	116	25	0	1
Shrimp	4 oz.	99	17	0	1
Venison	4 oz.	158	30	0	3
Red Snapper	4 oz.	128	26	0	2
Deli Roast Beef	4 oz.	200	8	2	1
Deli Ham	4 oz.	145	21	2	6
Lamb Choice	4 oz.	191	28	0	8

Grains/Breads/ Pasta	Serving Size	Calories	Protein (g)	Carbs (g)	Fat (g)
Oatmeal	1/2 cup dry	145	6	25	2
Whole-Grain Cereal	3/4 cup	110	3	24	1
Whole Wheat Bread	1 slice	19	3	13	1
Plain Bagel	1	195	7	38	1
English Muffin	1	127	5	25	1
Whole Wheat Pita	1	170	6	35	2

Grains/Breads/ Pasta (cont)	Serving Size	Calories	Protein (g)	Carbs (g)	Fat (g)
Flour Tortilla, 8-inch	1	145	4	25	3
Corn Tortilla	1	58	2	12	1
White Rice	1 cup cooked	205	4	44	1
Brown Rice	1 cup cooked	216	5	45	2
Wild Rice	1 cup cooked	166	7	35	1
Couscous	1 cup cooked	176	6	36	1
Macaroni	1 cup cooked	197	7	40	1
Spaghetti	1 cup cooked	197	7	40	1
Bulgur	1 cup cooked	151	6	34	1
Bran Muffin	1	160	4	36	1
Sourdough bread	1 slice	69	2	13	1
Whole Wheat Crackers	5	89	2	14	3
Whole Wheat Pretzels	1 oz.	103	3	23	1

Fruit	Serving Size	Calories	Protein (g)	Carbs (g)	Fat (g)
Cantaloupe	1 cup	55	1	13	0
Strawberries	1 cup	46	1	11	0
Blueberries	1 cup	81	1	20	0
Apple	1	81	1	21	0
Orange	1	64	1	16	0
Grapefruit	½	37	1	9	0
Banana	1	109	1	28	0
Kiwi	1	46	1	11	0
Plum	1	36	1	9	0

Fruit (cont)	Serving Size	Calories	Protein (g)	Carbs (g)	Fat (g)
Peach	1	42	1	11	0
Nectarine	1	67	1	16	0
Apricots	3	50	1	12	0
Grapes	1 cup	114	1	28	0
Raisins	¼ cup	109	1	29	0
Pear	1	98	1	25	0
Pineapple	1	76	1	19	0
Orange Juice	1 cup	112	1	26	0
Avocado	1/4	77	1	3	0
Watermelon	1	49	1	11	0
Raspberries	1 cup	60	1	14	0

Vegetables	Serving Size	Calories	Protein (g)	Carbs (g)	Fat (g)
Broccoli Florets	1 cup	20	2	4	0
Bell Pepper	1 cup chopped	40	1	10	0
Onion	1 cup chopped	61	2	14	0
Tomato	1 lg.	38	2	8	0
Asparagus	4 spears	15	1	3	0
Collard Greens	1 cup	11	1	3	0
Spinach	1 cup	7	1	1	0
Eggplant	1/2 cup	1	1	3	0
Sweet potato	1	117	2	28	0
Potato	1 medium	120	3	28	0
Carrot	1	31	1	7	0
Green Peas	1/2 cup	67	4	12	0
Corn	1/2 cup	89	3	21	0

Vegetables (cont)	Serving Size	Calories	Protein (g)	Carbs (g)	Fat (g)
Zucchini	1 cup shredded	14	1	4	0
Garlic	1 clove	4	1	1	0
Tomato Juice	1 cup	46	2	11	0
Tomato Sauce	1/2 cup	37	2	9	0
Romaine lettuce	1 cup shredded	9	1	1	0
Cucumber	1 cup	14	1	3	0
Mushrooms	1 cup	18	2	3	0
Cauliflower	1 cup	25	2	5	0
Green Beans	1/2 cup	22	1	5	0
Artichoke	1	60	4	13	0
Salsa	1/2 cup	29	1	6	0

Milk/Egg Products	Serving Size	Calories	Protein (g)	Carbs (g)	Fat (g)
Egg, Large	1	75	6	1	5
Egg White	1	17	4	1	0
Egg Substitute	1/4 cup	53	8	1	2
1% Cottage Cheese	1/2 cup	82	14	3	1
Cheddar Cheese	1 oz.	49	7	1	2
Non-Fat Yogurt	8 oz.	127	13	17	1
Non-Fat Milk	1 cup	86	8	12	1
Raw Tofu	3.5 oz.	144	16	4	9
Swiss Cheese	1 slice	33	5	2	2

Legumes	Serving Size	Calories	Protein (g)	Carbs (g)	Fat (g)
Soybeans	1/2 cup	149	14	9	8
Lentils	1/2 cup	115	9	20	1
Black Beans	1/2 cup	114	8	20	1
Kidney Beans	1/2 cup	112	8	20	1
Baby Lima Beans	1/2 cup	115	7	21	1

Nuts/Seeds	Serving Size	Calories	Protein (g)	Carbs (g)	Fat (g)
Peanut Butter Natural	2 Tbsp	210	8	6	16
Walnuts	1 oz.	172	7	3	16
Peanuts	1 oz.	140	5	11	10
Flaxseeds	3 Tbsp	166	7	6	14

Hormone imbalances and stress buildup can lead to *decades* of demeaning, low-vitality, inferior living. In practice, "Reclaim 24" means that once you alter your habits for the better and get your hormones rebalanced, you will benefit 24 hours a day … even in your sleep! In doing so, you will "turn the clock back" to times you feared might be lost to you forever! And looking into your mirror will become a pleasure instead of a reason to wince.

It means reclaiming your life and youthful vitality. And it means maintaining your ability to provide not only for yourself but also for your children, your mate, and others who must depend on you to keep them "out from the cold."

Reclaim 24 is *the science of staying young, no matter what the calendar says!* There is no good reason for life to take a downward turn after you leave your 20's.

Index